Certified Christ-based Counselor's Handbook

▪ The Process of Being Made Whole ▪

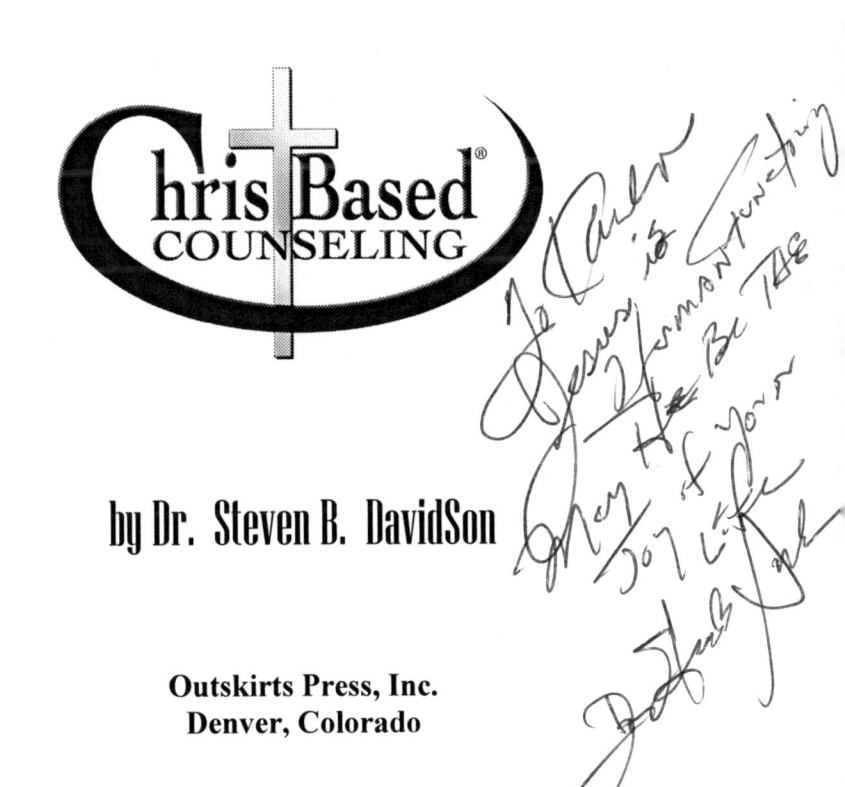

Christ Based COUNSELING

by Dr. Steven B. Davidson

Outskirts Press, Inc.
Denver, Colorado

The opinions expressed in this manuscript are solely the opinions of the author and do not represent the opinions or thoughts of the publisher.

Certified Christ-based Counselor's Handbook
The Process of Being Made Whole
All Rights Reserved
Copyright © 2005 Dr. Steven B. DavidSon
vr 1.2

This book may not be reproduced, transmitted, or stored in whole or in part by any means, including graphic, electronic, or mechanical without the express written consent of the publisher except in the case of brief quotations embodied in critical articles and reviews.

Biblical references: The Authorized Version of the King James Version is in the public domain.
"Scripture quotations taken from the New American Standard Bible, Copyright 1960, 1962, 1963, 1968, 1971, 1972, 1973, 1975, 1977, 1995 by the Lockman Foundation Used by permission."
(www.Lockman.org)
Scripture quotations marked NLT or New Living Translation are taken from the Holy Bible, New Living Translation, copyright © 1996. Used by permission of Tyndale House Publishers, Inc., Wheaton, Illinois 60189, all rights reserved."

Outskirts Press
http://www.outskirtspress.com

ISBN: 1-932672-40-0

Outskirts Press and the "OP" logo are trademarks belonging to Outskirts Press, Inc.

Printed in the United States of America

About the Author

Dr. Steven B. DavidSon is founder of the National Association of Certified Christ-based Counselors in its 12th year. He designed the Christ-based Counseling model, but refers to Jesus as the origin, architect, and empowerment of the Christ-based Counseling framework. Thousands have taken advantage of his works in areas such as marriage, homosexuality, depression, anorexia and bulimia, child discipline, and addiction just to name a few. His Christ-based model is far superior to Christian counseling where often psychology is employed under the guise of sprinkled Scripture text. Dr. Paul Carlin the director and founder of Therapon Institute calls Dr. DavidSon's works the most profound Christ-based concepts he has ever witnessed.

Table of Contents

Christ-based Counseling (CBC), The Model

The Antecedent Commission	3
The Approach	7
The Theology vs. Psychology Debate	9
The Objective of Christ-based Counseling	11
The Process of Being Made Whole	13
Scientific Evidence	17
The Issue of Hermeneutics	19
Organic Problems	25
The Dynamics of Choice	27
Motivation	31
The Will of God	35
Life Transformation Not Behavior Modification	41
Beyond Heredity and Environment	45
Hard Core Cases	49
The Unparalleled Sufficiency of Christ-based Counseling	55
The Process of Being Made Whole (Counseling Primer/Orientation)	57
College of Professional Studies Course	63

Christ-based Counseling, Illustrated

Preparation and Distinction	73

Marriage, Divorce and the Believer

The Divorce Phenomena	77
The Formative Years	79
A Study on Christian Marriage	87
A Study on Divorce and the Christian	95
The Exception Clause, Limiting and Liberating	99
Times of Struggle Revisited	111
For Better or For Worse	121
A Matter of Repentance	135
Final Thoughts	143
Notes	145
Bibliography	147

Liberation and Deliverance Therapy

Preface	153
L&D Introduction	157
Addictiveness and Addiction a Biblical Perspective (Part I)	159
Description of Addiction and Addictiveness	159
Causes for Addiction and Addictiveness	160
Dynamics of Liberation (Part II)	165
Cry for Liberation	165
God's Purpose	166
God Calls an Intercessor	167
God Declares the Time of Liberation	168
God Assaults the Benefactor of the Addiction	169
Relapse Amidst Recovery	169
Personal Liberation, Interdiction and Duration	170
Dynamics of Deliverance (Part III)	177
A Period of Praise	178
Odious Memories	178
Negated Prayers	179
L&D Programming for Believers Suffering Addictions	181
Program Activities	181
Program Duration	183
Sessions	183
Program Reports	183
Terminating L&D	183
L&D Assessment Guide	185
L&D Assessment	185
L&D Assessment Follow-up	203

Joy Therapy
Overcoming Depression   223

Appendix
Marriage Enhancement Program   241
Actual Christ-based Counseling Notes for a Family   261
(Concerning Families with Step-children, and Teenaged or Adult Children)

Christ-based Counseling (CBC)
The Model

The Antecedent Commission

Like the ancient oath in the medical sciences, Christ-based Counseling's origin is in the "Antecedent Commission" of Jesus Christ (Matthew 10:1,7; Mark 6:7,12-13; Luke 9:1,6). The term, Great Commission is familiar to believers worldwide. It is the universal call to make disciples (Matthew 28:19-20). The Great Commission requires the creation of disciples based on all that Jesus taught and demonstrated.

The Antecedent Commission provides descriptive detail of what "all" in the Great Commission entails. The Antecedent Commission illustrates the specific plagues of mankind, which must be overcome. This is the first commission and continues to be the keystone of Christ-based Counseling. Jesus sends his disciples forth as follows:

And having summoned His twelve disciples, He gave them authority over unclean spirits, to cast them out, and to heal every kind of disease and every kind of sickness... And as you go, preach, saying, The kingdom of heaven is at hand.
(Matthew 10:1,7)

These words of Jesus stand as the purpose for the Christ-based Counselor's ministry. Jesus clearly identifies the three plagues upon mankind: (1) spiritual assault, (2) deteriorating physical and mental health, (3) social and relational degradation. Jesus addresses every issue facing mankind when he uses the terms, "every kind" of disease AND "every kind" of sickness. However, Jesus is intentional in all that He does. The first task is to defeat agents of "every kind" of sickness in the spiritual realm. The Christ-based Counselor understands that there is a major and determining spiritual component to all other maladies faced by believers. This spiritual target must be addressed while dealing with any other issue, or using any other therapeutic modes for healing God's people. The spiritual weapons of faith, God's Word, and prayer are not secondary instruments for therapy (Ephesians 6:16-18). These are the primary instruments of therapy for God's people. Medical sciences are secondary, and socio-psycho practices where appropriate follow. The Christ-based Counselor believes that the medical field is an obvious benefit. Christ-based Counselors believe in the progressive provision principle. That is, as God provides man the wherewithal to provide for himself, God no longer provides in that area. This includes any area of need concerning health or otherwise.

We can see this principle in numerous examples throughout the Bible. As early as Noah, we see God providing for him and his family. It is understood that the ark carried enough sustenance within the ark. But once the land was dry, they no longer had to eat from the food on the ark (Genesis 9:1-3). Likewise, when the Hebrews entered the promise land it was no longer necessary for God to provide manna by day. They could retrieve and grow their own food (Joshua 5:12). Once it was necessary for the priest to intercede for the people. However, God provides a marvelous provision in Jesus Christ so all believers can approach God personally (Hebrews 4:14-16). The old system is no longer necessary.

Today, humanity's medical therapies are extraordinary. A broken arm, or life threatening disease, man has designed medicinal therapies that are highly successful. The Apostle Paul prescribes a medicinal therapy for Timothy,

> *No longer drink water exclusively, but use a little wine*
> *for the sake of your stomach and your frequent ailments*
> *(I Timothy 5:23).*

The Apostle James also recognized the wisdom of medicinal therapy. He directed elders as follows:

> *Is anyone among you sick? Let him call for the elders of the church, and let them pray over him, anointing him with oil in the name of the Lord*
> *(James 5:14).*

While there are persons who see the oil figuratively as the Holy Spirit, the fact is that James is talking about literal-oil that has medicinal characteristics. Notice that the therapy is to be provided in the name of the Lord. If he intended that the oil was actually the Holy Spirit, there would be no need to apply the oil in the name of the Lord. The term, in the name of the Lord was customarily used to "sanctify" a process that would otherwise be quite natural. Again, no such sanctification process would be needed if the oil was the Holy Spirit. Both cases (i.e., Paul, James) demonstrate that these pillars of the New Testament movement respected the value of medicinal helps. Since they also had the ability to heal people with their physical touch, this also demonstrates God's progressive provision. There was no need for a miracle-of-healing when all that was necessary was good sense, a little wine, or oil. Prayer, of course is always applied regardless of the circumstances (i.e., miracle, or medicinal therapy).

Therefore, Christ-based Counselors work closely with other professionals seeking their perspective.

However, the caution flag must be lifted for pharmaceutical therapy of all types, and particularly any dealing with psychic functioning. And any non-medicinal therapy dealing with behavior, attitude, disposition, internal principles, mores and similar functioning must meet the litmus test of God's Word for believers. This is the area where humanity has not progressed. Humanity continues to be adulterous, incestuous, deceitful, inconsistent, irresponsible, anti-social, self-destructive, seditious, and the like. While the progenitors of the psycho-socio sciences have tried to understand man's plight, no one understands mankind like Jesus Christ. Stated simply, Christ-based Counseling is a "root" cause approach. This is the critical path of any therapy designed for issues facing the believer. All human illnesses (physical, psychological, social, etc.) have a spiritual root. Therein lies the significance of Paul's wrap-up of the human issues he covered in Ephesians. The fact is, it could be called a wrap-up of all his writings concerning the root cause of the human condition. Paul stated, "we wrestle not against flesh and blood..." (Ephesians 6:12). Thus:

<u>This is the principal call and cause for Christ-based Counseling.</u>

The Approach

The National Association of Certified Christ-based Counselors' (NACCBC) counseling approach is characterized as Christ-based Counseling. A Christ-based Counseling approach is appropriate, not only because the objective is to guide the counselee in a manner that will improve his or her Christian walk; but also because Jesus Christ Himself introduces the model for all of the concepts or principles.

Currently there exists a multitude of approaches to Christian counseling. The term, Christian Counseling is rightfully under suspicion. In fact there are those who even propose that the term Christian Counseling is somehow anti-Christian, notwithstanding all of the arguments which seem to exist. The Christ-based Counseling approach uses those resources available to all believers in the body of Christ, viz. (1) the Bible, which is the existing body of information familiar to the Christ-based Counselor, and (2) the counselor's virtue of care.

This sounds very simple. However, this is not an effort to over simplify an extremely technical field. Furthermore, this is not an agenda to insinuate that specific educational programs are not necessary. NACCBC membership includes individuals with advanced degrees in the Christian counseling field, and social and medical sciences. However, the predominant principle in developing a counseling approach must be to use the power and authority available in the angelic dimension first, and the natural dimension secondarily.

The historic facts prove that well before the secular counseling disciplines were developed, people's lives were being transformed by their introduction to Jesus Christ, and this fact is as true today as in the past. In my estimation no other therapy, concept, approach, principle, et al. has dramatically changed lives as the Gospel. Neither the Church nor individual lives are dependent on any foundation other than Jesus Christ. Certainly, if a truth or concept is not against the Church, it can be perceived as a support. However, not even a support is required. The Church is Christ-sufficient.

Therefore, Christ-based Counseling relies on the fact that there is not one pathological, relational, or personal issue which exists that cannot be related to the life of Jesus Christ in the Bible. Identify the issues--drug and alcohol abuse, AIDS, incest, marital discord, sexual promiscuity, sexual molestation, perjury, larceny, extortion, gossip, idolatry, et al.--all are covered. Contributing factors such as heredity, and environmental concerns are also covered. These facts will be demonstrated later.

The Theology vs. Psychology Debate

While the Christian counseling community argues over the issues of integrating psychology and theology, Satan is having a field day. Believers do not need an aura of uncertainty lingering over the persons most responsible for their spiritual well being (e.g., pastors, elders, presbyters, etc.). The Christ-based Counselor must continue to discover methods of integrating the personality of Jesus Christ into the believer's life. So at this point we leave the continuing saga of who's right, and who's wrong to those who have been mired in this predicament. While we are extremely familiar with a number of these Christian practitioners' works, we will purposely omit names in order to avoid ostracism or fraternization. We have no intention of spending any more than this paragraph addressing the theology/psychology quagmire. We are too busy trying to change lives through Jesus Christ.

The Objective of Christ-based Counseling

Every writer in the counseling field has provided an opinion on the objective of Christian counseling. Most of the opinions are scholarly, and even Biblically acceptable. Christ-based Counseling's objective for counseling is not new. We believe that we cannot improve upon what Jesus Christ stated numerous times as He sought to do the will of His Father. Focused on Jesus' ministry, we see our major purpose in the counseling arena as:

Providing guidance for believers to do the will of the Father.

The Process of Being Made Whole

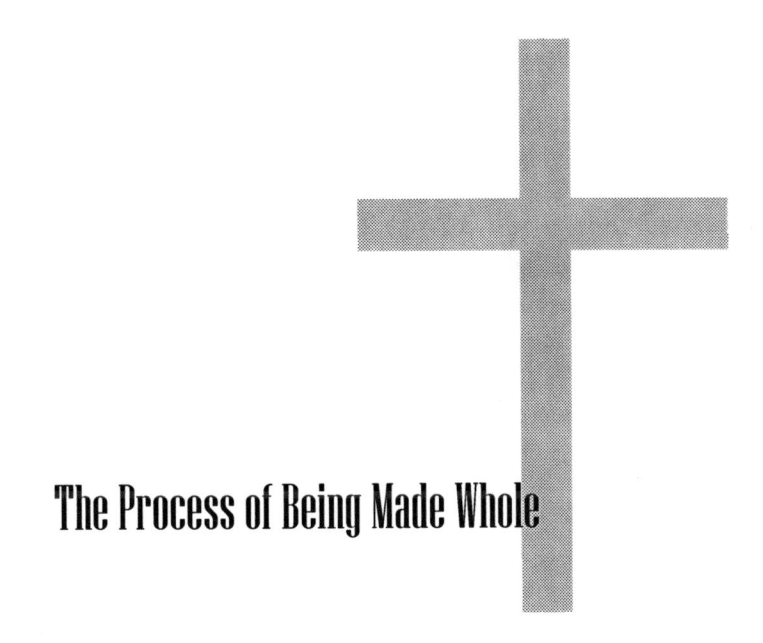

A number of Christian counseling books possess highly elaborate diagrams and schematics of the cognitive processes, social interaction postulates, existential hypotheses, and similar systems. They are scholarly, demonstrative of the technical sophistication possessed by the clinicians, and intellectually challenging. Some of these books even have spiritual value. Since the Christian counselee can present a complex web of difficulties to the Christ-based Counselor, it may appear appropriate to offer approaches as intricate as the problems.

Christ-based Counseling's theory is not a theory at all. Christ-based Counseling espouses a spiritual process designed to make the person whole, and thereby satisfying the counseling objective. All non-organic problems confronted in the counseling experience are appropriately resolved when the believer implements the following principles which we define as the Process of Being Made Whole.

The Process

1. The counselee must be born again (John 3:3; 3:11-12).

2. The counselee must be presented balanced Biblical information to make the right decision or decisions (Matt. 4:6-7).

3. The counselee must possess the degree of faith needed to implement the properties of the decision or decisions (Mark 4:24).

4. The counselee must be committed to spiritual development while experiencing the preliminary results of the decision or decisions (Luke 21:1-4).

5. The counselee must be provided the practical support to experience the joy of the decision or decisions (Mark 8:1-3; 2:4).

6. The counselee must continue the process in spite of the final outcome of the decision or decisions (John 15:4-7; 10-11).

7. Strategic and persistent prayer mobilizes the powers in the angelic realm with impact in the counselee's physical realm (Luke 11:1-8; Luke 18:1-8).

The Process Explained

The counselee must be born again: This part of the process should not need an explanation.

Balanced Biblical information: The use of Biblical illustrations must be acceptable for the purposes intended. This is discussed at length under "The Issue of Hermeneutics."

The degree of faith needed: In practically every case in the New Testament model, faith is a required factor of the process of "making whole." The greater the dilemma, the more resolute one's exercise of faith must be.

Commitment to spiritual development: The believer must be determined to grow spiritually beyond his or her present stature.

Practical support: There must be a support system including the pastor, elders, and other believers who will provide counseling sessions, prayer, fellowship, encouragement, and other assistance.

Continuing the process: As long as the condition exists, the counselee must remain committed to the Process. There should always be some level of the Process on-going in the counselee's life regardless of the circumstances.

Strategic and persistent prayer: The counselee must pray about the specific counseling issue, persistently.

Scientific Evidence

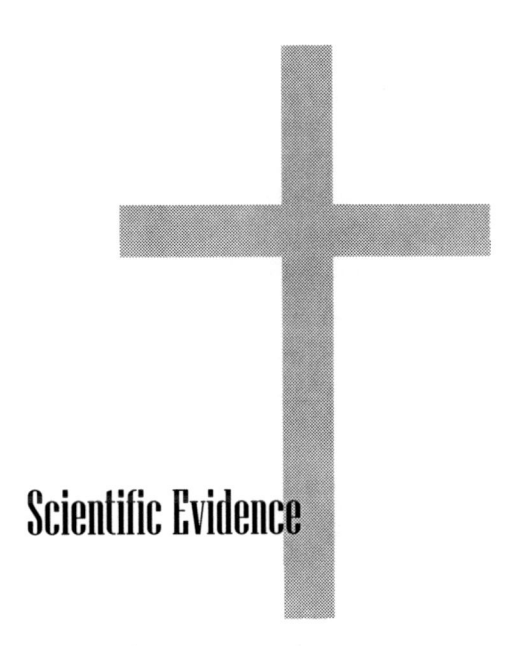

This section is for the believers who need to satisfy clinical parameters to accept the validity of the truths in the Process. For the readers who know that the process above is true, you can move to the next section.

As stated previously, all non-organic problems confronted in the counseling experience are appropriately resolved when the believer practices "The Process of Making Whole." Since the word, "all" will not be accepted by the counselor with a scientific mental paradigm, perhaps a quantitative measurement would be more appropriate. Therefore, 100% of all non-organic counseling problems are appropriately resolved. Please note the use of the adverb, appropriately. Eventually, all problems are resolved, regardless of the method used to address the counselee's concern (i.e., through death, dissolution, imprisonment, drug abuse, etc.). However, what the Christ-based Counselor endeavors to accomplish is a solution that will meet the Christ-based Counseling objective stated previously.

Nevertheless, for the scientific brethren who prefer statistical facts and case studies, I invite you to conduct your most critical analysis of the books of Matthew, Mark, Luke, and John. I believe that you will discover a 100% success rate of the case studies in the Gospels. If this is not satisfactory, I cannot do any better, and I will not try.

However, I recommend for your homework that you read 100 times or more per day "The Process of Being Made Whole," and take the necessary steps personally to actualize each constituent of the process. After completing the "Process," conduct your critical analysis of Matthew, Mark, Luke, and John again. If you have done as counseled, you will discover a 100% success rate of the numerous case studies. Furthermore, do not forget to add your contribution to the statistics, and include your testimony to the catalog of case studies. Now that you have completed this exercise, you may proceed to the next section.

The Issue of Hermeneutics

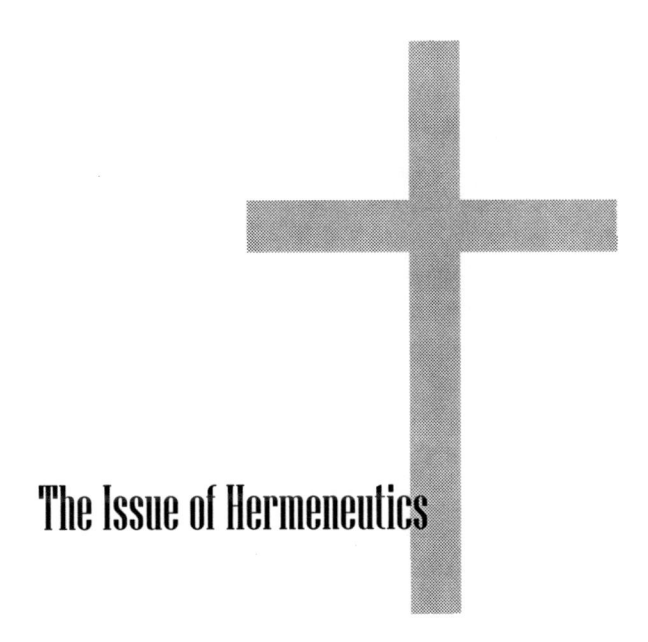

Once you have accepted "The Process of Being Made Whole," you may encounter difficulties understanding how the life of Jesus Christ can be related to many of the issues common to counseling sessions today. The New Testament does not provide literal advice on a number of these issues, and acceptable principles of hermeneutics simply will not allow the application of Biblical text to address them.

Biblical interpretation becomes an issue of great concern for all of us who desire to honor the specific conditions addressed by any body of text presented in Scripture. Developing counseling applications or models from the four Gospels could be construed as manipulation of Scripture beyond the limits of acceptability. That is, when a counselee's condition is related to an event in the Gospels other than the specific circumstances cited in the Biblical account, this would appear to violate principles of acceptable interpretation.

For the purpose of this document the use of the terms models, principles, or applications are interchangeable unless they are defined differently.

Rules Governing a Christ-based Counselor's Application

For the purpose of clarity, a brief explanation of the differences between interpretation and application is required. According to conservative scholarship, acceptable INTERPRETATION of any text must be limited to the specific conditions and situations a given body of text discusses. The APPLICATION of the text is the process of applying or making relative the interpreted text to contemporary experiences (i.e., as long as the contemporary experience is the same).

We respond to this extremely serious matter with the following:

Rules to Govern the Christ-based Counselor's Application of Biblical Truths

1. The counselor must consider the prevailing Biblical circumstances or events, including all of the related issues.
2. When relating to the life of Jesus Christ, the scope of interpretation in a specific area is too narrow if it is not interpreted from a synergistic perspective.
3. With all due respect to the theologians, interpreters, and etymologists, the Christ-based Counselor's interpretation of the Gospels must be evaluated in light of Jesus' explanations of His teachings. Matthew 16:1-12 (also see Mark 8:14-21), represents an example of Jesus' implicit interpretational standards.

And the Pharisees and Sadducees came up, and testing Him asked Him to show them a sign from heaven.

And the disciples came to the other side and had forgotten to take bread.

And Jesus said to them, "Watch out and beware of the leaven of the Pharisees and Sadducees."

And they began to discuss among themselves, saying, "It is because we took no bread."

But Jesus, aware of this, said, "You men of little faith, why do you discuss among yourselves that you have no bread?"

> *"Do you not yet understand or remember the five loaves of the five thousand, and how many baskets you took up?"*
>
> *"Or the seven loaves of the four thousand, and how many large baskets you took up?*
>
> *"How is it that you do not understand that I did not speak to you concerning bread? But beware of the leaven of the Pharisees and Sadducees."*
>
> *Then they understood that He did not say to beware of the leaven of bread, but of the teaching of the Pharisees and Sadducees.*

Jesus begins His conversation with the disciples by issuing a warning about the teachings of the Pharisees and Sadducees. However, due to the disciples' lack of understanding, another issue surfaces. The secondary issue is that they are not able to understand the meaning of the primary issue (i.e., the warning about the Pharisees and Sadducees). This misunderstanding occurs for the following reasons: (1) they were mentally incapacitated by their own sense of forgetfulness; (2) they did not consider that Jesus was speaking in the context of his exchange with the Pharisees and Sadducees; (3) they did not use their insight of the abilities and personality of Jesus when they attempted to understand His warning. Obviously, one loaf of bread to be shared among the disciples was not a problem for Jesus Who could feed thousands with a few loaves.

Clearly, they recognized that Jesus was using some kind of symbolism. Their discussion did not even include the Pharisees or Sadducees. If they would have used the first rule (see "Rules to Govern a Christ-based Counselor's Application"), they would have realized that he was speaking about the Pharisees and Sadducees, and people like them. They also knew that some aspect of the warning was to be taken literally. This fact is demonstrated by their discussion in verse 7, "And they began to discuss among themselves, saying, 'It is because we took no bread.'" If they would have used Rules 2 and 3, they would have recognized that literal bread was not Jesus' concern.

Below, you will find excerpts from commentators concerning the disciples' misinterpretation, and what Jesus taught concerning the interpretation of His teachings:

The disciples failed at first to understand what Jesus meant. They thought he referred to literal leaven.[1] Jesus warns his followers to beware of this teaching. But the reference to the 2 feedings, or 5 and 4 thousand respectively, is presented as though it were self explanatory, which it is not. Matthew's implication is that the feeding stories contain some teaching of the truth, which His followers are supposed to grasp.[2]

The permeating evil influence of these determined opponents of Christ (i.e., Pharisees and Sadducees) is the point involved. Yet the disciples, embarrassed at their oversight, failed to grasp the symbolism.[3]

He took it ill that they should be so little acquainted with his way of preaching. Then understood they what he meant. Christ teaches by the Spirit of wisdom in the heart, opening the understanding to the Spirit of revelation in the Word.[4]

If the disciples had reflected on the fact that concern with reference to bread for a small company, though understandable, was totally out of place on the basis of the fact that Jesus with a few bread-cakes had twice fed thousands, with plenty of bread left on both occasions, their minds would have turned in a different direction in attempting to interpret the Master's warning with respect to "the yeast of the Pharisees and Sadducees.[5]"

The Christ-based Counselor's System of Application

Based on the text (Matt. 16:1-12), and the "Rules Governing a Christ-based Counselor's Application," a brief paraphrase of the spirit and intent of what Jesus states to the disciples in regards to understanding his teachings can be rendered as follows:

I should not have to tell you everything. Whenever you are evaluating my instructions, think. You must apply the principles I teach you, based on the circumstances,

what you have witnessed in regards to my life, and who
I AM.

Given the aforementioned, establishing a construct for Christ-based Counseling using the Gospel does not violate acceptable hermeneutical practices. It may indeed violate systems devised by men, but it does not violate the interpretational system authorized by Jesus Christ, Himself. Nevertheless, in our efforts to impress upon the Christ-based Counselor the critical nature of this area, we conclude this section by invoking an additional test designed carefully to guide the Christ-based Counselor through the maze of acceptable applications.

The Test of a Viable Counseling Application

Additionally, to employ the rules stated above, each application as defined must satisfy the elements of this test. Therefore, a counseling application relative to a body of text is viable when it satisfies the following:

1. The application is faithful to the spirit and intent of the text.
2. The application is consistent with the full scope of the attributes and the personality of Jesus Christ.
3. The application does not violate any other New Testament doctrine.
4. The counselor expresses to the counselee that it is an application based on the description above and is not to be understood as a strict interpretation. Given the Rules and Test, the models, application, or principles for any condition confronting Christ-based Counseling can be developed.

Organic Problems

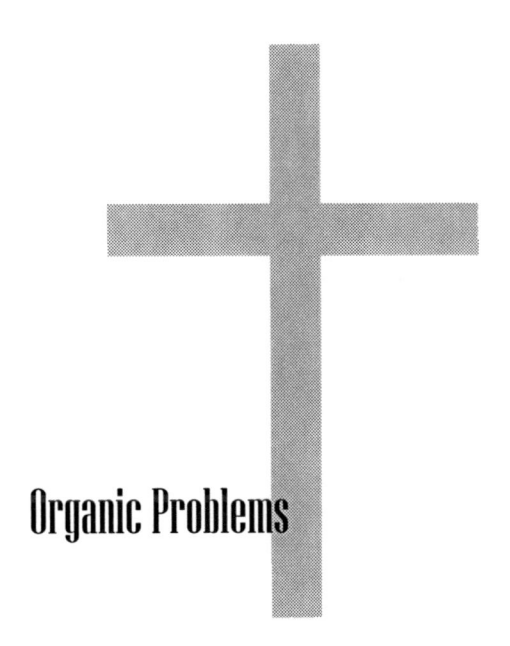

First, a definition of the term organic must be provided. The term organic means that the counselee possesses a disorder related to his or her physical anatomy or biochemical metabolism. When the counselee is a member of a medical plan or health maintenance organization, it is extremely accommodating to recommend him or her to a physician. However, without a medical plan the situation is not so clear. Even government medical facilities will accept only the most dire situations. In cases of this nature, the counselor must recommend the counselee with an official letter to a physician or care facility. The counselor must maintain the letter, and any response to the letter. The counselor continues as with any other counselee, remembering that Jesus also has a 100% success rate with organic problems

The Dynamics of Choice

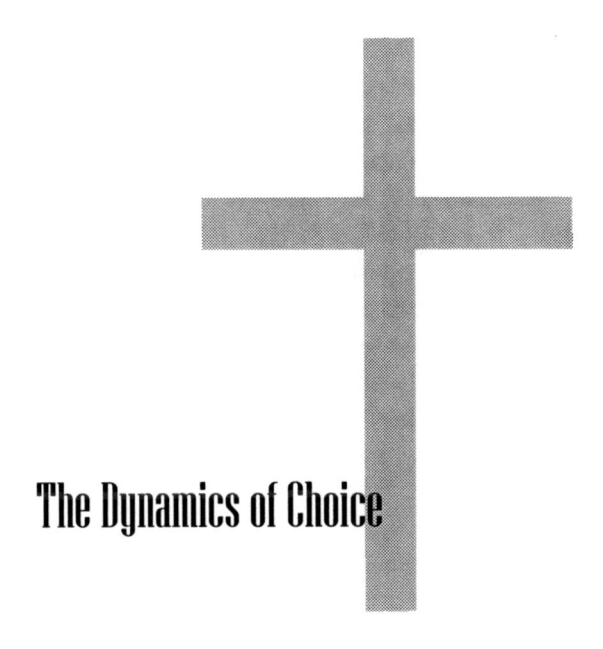

Typically, the counselee is faced with one or more alternatives and/or processes to resolve the issue facing the counselee. Once an individual is provided balanced Biblical counseling on the appropriate alternatives, how does the person actually choose and implement the right alternative?

There are a number of factors that can influence an individual's ability to implement the Biblical alternative. Where organic problems do not exist, the choice depends on what the individual believes to provide the best results.

Often the alternatives include remaining in the existing condition the counselee is seeking counsel to change.

Unfortunately, choosing the tangible, natural alternative is more preferable than the biblical, intangible alternative. The tangible alternative usually provides an immediate answer and short relief -- usually temporary. Since it already exists in some form, the tangible, natural alternative is also readily accepted.

The Biblical alternative represents a choice that will provide a more satisfactory and long lasting result. However, by its nature it is intangible from a physical or natural sense, and may even appear less attractive in the short term.

Concept vs. Reality Dilemma

To further understand the constituents of choice, the Christ-based Counselor must understand different stages of the believer's ability to bring Biblical principles into reality.

The believer suffers the dilemma of moving from knowing what is right to doing what is right. The Apostle Paul clearly describes the believer's condition in the Book of Romans, which prevents the believer from exercising Biblical principles in perfection.

Since the Bible is our primary book for Christ-based Counseling, I recommend a detailed study of Romans (i.e., Romans 7-9).

Nevertheless, the approach here is to discuss from a practical perspective why a counselee is not able to implement a Biblical decision (i.e., even when they possess the appropriate Biblical direction).

It is not the Christ-based Counseling position that there exist different categories of truth. However, truths are facilitated differently in an individual's life.

The believer's administration of truth can be characterized in two stages, Conceptual and Reality.

Truth Stages

The Conceptual Truth Stage is evident when the merits of a principle, event, or act are perceived in the mind as being acceptable and reliable. The Conceptual Truth Stage is usually fixed (i.e., unchangeable) unless the counselee is presented convincing information to disprove the Conceptual Truth.

The Reality Truth Stage occurs when the merits of a principle, event, or act are perceived in the mind as being acceptable and reliable, and decisions are made to implement the truth in spite of the perceived consequences. Unlike the Conceptual Truth Stage, the Reality Truth Stage is variable (i.e., fluctuates).

Whether or not an individual is able to move from the Concept Stage to Reality Stage depends on motivational factors, which are discussed later.

When the counselee accepts the Biblical principle as true (i.e., Conceptual Truth Stage), but determines that in reality it is not the best choice, the counselee is suffering from a Reality Truth Deficit.

There are numerous illustrations of these three factors (i.e., Conceptual Truth Stage, Reality Truth Stage, and Reality Truth Deficit). The following Biblical account demonstrates all three.

Biblical Illustration of the Stages of Choice

The occasion when Jesus was walking across the water (Matt.14:28-29) clearly illustrates the dynamics of choice. Mark's account is more descriptive in regards to Jesus' intentions as he proceeded across the water. Before beginning his "hydrotrek" He saw them struggling or toiling against the winds. He was going to walk past them on the way to the other side (Mark 6:48). Understandably, they were frightened when they saw him reasoning that it must be a spirit. However, one of the disciples (Peter) perceived that walking with Jesus was better than struggling in the boat -- if it was indeed Jesus.

All of the disciples had the same alternatives (i.e., stay in the boat, or walk with Jesus). They had to make their respective decisions based on what they believed would provide the best results. Speculatively, the other disciples may have entered the Conceptual Truth Stage. That is, they may have known conceptually that walking with Jesus on the water was a better choice than struggling in a boat, but they did not believe in the reality of such a choice (i.e., Reality Truth Deficit). The "stakes" were too high to try. As stated earlier, as with most counseling situations, one of the disciples alternatives was simply to remain in their existing condition (i.e., struggling in the boat). Excluding Peter, they decided to stay.

Reality Truth Deficit

Definitively, Peter entered the Conceptual Truth Stage and moved to the Reality Truth Stage. He believed conceptually that -- if indeed -- it was Jesus, he (Peter) would be given the ability to walk on water. He moved to the Reality Truth Stage when he asked Jesus' approval to walk on the water. Once he received approval, Peter began to walk upon the water (i.e., Reality Truth Stage).

However, one of the dynamics of entering the Reality Truth Stage is that as the individual (Peter) moves progressively in the Reality

Truth Stage, the threshold for Reality Truth Deficit grows proportionately. Therefore, the same level of Reality Truth that Peter began with on his first step had to be maintained.

Unfortunately, as Peter moved progressively, he suffered from Reality Truth Deficit. He began to believe that what he was doing was becoming less reliable (i.e., walking on water), and that the adverse consequences were potentially more reliable. Since the Reality Truth Stage is variable, Peter changed from the Reality Truth Stage to the Conceptual Truth Stage, and the Conceptual Truth Stage is fruitless in the believers life. Clearly, it was more dangerous for Peter to be wavering in the Reality Truth Stage than not to enter it at all. However, Jesus does save Peter as he begins to sink.

When Jesus enters the boat he reprimands the disciples for their unfaithfulness. Unfaithfulness is a personal declaration that following Jesus (i.e., Biblical principles) is not reliable in reality. Simply stated, God's principles are pretentious.

Motivation

Motivation is the actual impetus that ignites the counselee to implement the Biblical principle in Christ-based Counseling. Motivation is the sole domain of the Holy Spirit (John 16:13). The Holy Spirit invokes at least two types of motivation, Prodigal and Centurion. All other forms of Christ-based Counseling motivation are variations of these two.

So far the constituents of choice have been expounded. Additionally an explanation has been provided for why a believer selects an unbiblical alternative. However, it is common that believers who initially select an unbiblical alternative, ultimately turn to a Biblical alternative.

Prodigal Motivation

As with the disciples in the illustration above, the believer may accept a truth in concept, but implementing the truth is perceived as too costly. Therefore, the Biblical alternative is selected when suffering which results from the unbiblical alternative, exceeds the perceived suffering which would occur from selecting the Biblical alternative. This type of motivation is referred to as Prodigal Motivation. This type of motivation is named after the experience of the prodigal son in (Luke 15:11-24). The son's abject condition was necessary to inspire the young man to "come to himself" and decide to return to his father. Please note the son's evaluation process before he decided to return home. He concluded, "my father's servants eat better than this." The suffering resulting from the unbiblical decision to leave home, exceeded the perceived suffering of the Biblical alternative to stay home, or in this case to return home.

Prodigal Motivation is typically required for believers who are spiritually paralyzed by sin, or any other condition requiring the most severe application of motivation.

Christ-based Counseling
The Dynamics of Choice
(In counseling we help people make the right or best choices)

Y (Life)
VICTORY

(Matt. 10:39; Matt. 16:25; Mk. 8:35; Lk. 9:24)
You Save, You Lose
You Lose, You Save

0 ——— (Decision Time Line)

• Runs out of money
• Hires Himself to Outsider
• Desired Swine's food
• Comes to HIMSELF
(Suffering resulting from the psychological decision exceeds the perceived suffering from the biblical decision)

SORROW
S (Death)

——— Psychological Decision
— — Christ-based Decision

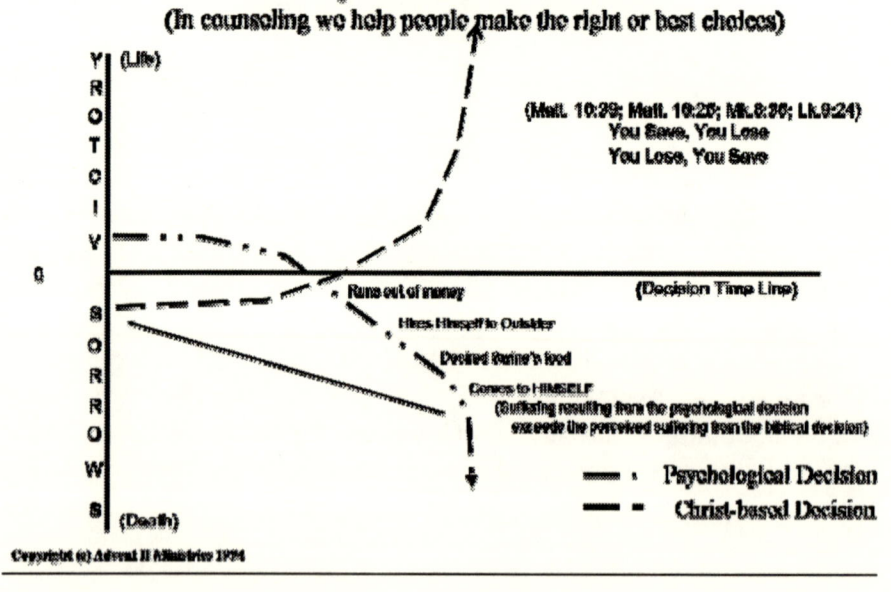

Copyright (c) Advent II Ministries 1994

This graphic illustrates why people make wrong decisions. As in the case with the prodigal son, he made his decision on what he saw as most advantageous. The dashed line begins below the Decision Time Line. This is where he perceives himself to be. If he can get the money from his father, and live as he pleases he begins or moves to a more satisfying life. This is depicted by the dot-dashed line where it appears to be more satisfying and victorious. However, during the course of time his decision begins to go "down-slope." Comparatively, if he had made the appropriate decision, the results would have led to a victorious life as depicted by the dashed-line. Humans are self-gratification oriented, and humans are intelligent. He used his natural, psychological thinking (I Corinthians 2:14-15). The term natural man in the Greek is psuchekos (i.e., or psychological man). Once the results from the decision of his natural thinking caused more suffering than his original condition, he came to himself. He returned to his father. This is depicted by the arrow pointing back to his original starting place.

Centurion Motivation

Centurion Motivation is based on the example of the centurion (Matt. 8:5-13) who reasoned that by virtue of Jesus' character and position, He (Jesus) had only to give the command to heal his (i.e., the centurions) servant.

The most virtuous source of motivation is God's Word, and acting upon His Word represents the greatest act of faith and trust. Jesus commented "I have not found in all of the house of Israel one with greater faith." Needless to say, the centurion's servant was healed before he arrived home. Centurion Motivation is typically demonstrated by persons who desire the most progressive, and miraculous manifestations of God's work in their lives.

The Will of God

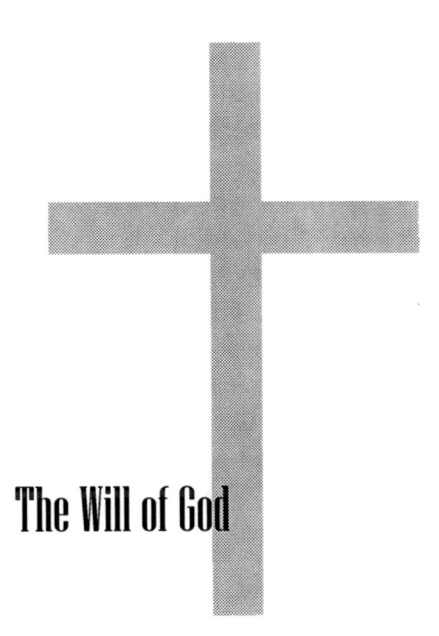

One of the most tenuous concepts in the believer's life is determining the will of God. A believer's personal understanding of God's will in any particular situation can be represented by mystical symbolism and correlations, dreams, curious life experiences, deja vu, hearing voices, and other similar occurrences.

Often the counselee desires to know God's will in situations such as mate selection, careers, ministry vocations, selection of a local church and many similar choices. Typically, as the significance of the choice increases, the tendency to seek God's will becomes more apparent.

Rarely will a believer seek God's will to determine what to prepare for the morning's breakfast. However, it is more likely that the same believer when confronted with the choice to select a mate, or change ministries will seek God's will in the matter.

There are five factors to be considered when an individual is attempting to understand God's will.

The Word Factor

The first of the five factors is the Word Factor. There are a number of decisions in life that are clearly explained by Biblical principles. A wife does not have to ask God whether she should forgive her husband who has repented of his sin (i.e., he is both remorseful, and exhibits a behavioral change). The teenaged son does not have to seek God's will of whether or not he should lie to his parents. The offended believer does not have to ask God whether he should approach the believer who was the source of the offense. It is preposterous to wonder about God's will in regards to an unmarried believer who desires a married person. Similarly, it is absolute nonsense to believe that special circumstances exist which allows an individual to violate strict Biblical principles. The guidance for these issues as well as others are stated in Biblical teachings.

The Personal Factor

This is perhaps the most misunderstood, and overlooked factor of the five. The believer has the tendency of seeing everything in black or white. That is, God is so static He does not have the ability to provide more than two alternatives. Given this outlook, the believer must wait for the right alternative to be revealed. It never occurs to the believer that while he or she is asking God "which way shall I go," God is responding, "which way do you desire to go." Nevertheless there are times when waiting for an event to occur is required, which shall be discussed later.

God has provided the framework for the believer to make decisions, and He is not going to get involved in minutia. This is not to say that he does not care about the minutia. God has provided the believer with the capabilities to determine the details, and He will not violate the individual's sovereignty.

Most believers practice this reality on a daily basis. Again, using the analogy of preparing breakfast, the believer may ask God what to prepare on a special occasion. However, it would be unusual to ask God each day what to prepare for breakfast. Even if a believer did ask God each day what to prepare for breakfast, the final decision would be based on the stock in the cabinets, available funds for food, other sources of food, and the believer's ability to prepare the food. More importantly if the believer does not become involved in deciding what to eat and the effort to prepare the food, the believer will not eat that day.

The believer must use this same approach to making other decisions in life. As long as the need or desire does not interfere or violate other Biblical principles the choice should be considered within the realm of the believers desire.

However, the believer must also be willing to make the commitment to possess the necessary resources and/or abilities to bring the desire or need into reality.

Biblical Illustration of the Personal Factor

There are a number of Christ-based illustrations of the personal factor, but since we have previously discussed Peter's experience of walking on the water, it is convenient to continue with his experience.

When Peter saw Jesus he desired to walk to Him (Jesus). This was not an issue that violated any principle of God. Neither did Jesus ask or suggest for Peter to walk on the water. Also it was not necessary for Peter to walk on the water. Often believers are convinced that God only provides the believer with what the believer needs. Peter "desired" to walk on the water, and Jesus granted Peter's "desire." However, Peter would have to possess or develop the personal requirements to walk on the water. Peter needed a consistent level of faith to bring his desire into reality. Therefore, the believer should not expect God to honor a request without the believer's participation. The believer must be willing to possess or develop the abilities to fulfill his or her role in seeing the request materialize in reality.

Finally, there are occasions when the believer can clearly see the will of God, but desires a different direction. The Christ-based illustrations of this are numerous, but the most convincing is Jesus' prayer at Gethsamene.

Again, this example is in regards to personal choices, and not moral or otherwise Scriptural issues. Believers can infer from the prayer of Jesus that God does provide the believer with alternatives. Jesus prayed "let this cup pass over me." Jesus desired an alternative to the one He was encountering. Regardless of how the believer interprets "cup," the bottom line is that Jesus desired something different from what he perceived to be developing. Please note that Jesus asks for His request. Without any doubt Jesus knew that His time was near. He clearly stated to the disciples that His time had come, and He knew it was the will of His Father (John 12:23; Mark 14:41). However, according to His own teaching he asked "whatsoever" He desired (Matt. 21:22; John 14:13; 15:16; 16:23). In this case he asked that the cup (i.e., experience) be altered. Too often the believer dilutes the request to what he or she believes will be acceptable. Jesus instructs us to ask for whatsoever, and confirms this indicating that if earthly (evil) father's give good gifts, how much "more" will our Father in heaven give to those who ask him (Matt. 7:11; Luke 11:13).

If Jesus is the perfect son of God who completely understands the Father, then we learn from His experience that God is open to suggestions.

Not My Will Thy Will

Since Jesus knew the will of the Father, He (Jesus) made his request ancillary to the will of His Father. In this situation, Jesus is requesting a change to what He knows is the absolute will of the Father. Therefore, Jesus has to wait for the answer.

The answer is revealed when He is kissed by His betrayer and taken captive. The believer should always subordinate one's personal desire to the Father's will.

The Faith Factor

Regardless of how well the believer is able to understand the will of God, there is always a specter of the unknown involved when determining what His will is. The believer satisfies the unknown aspect of desire fulfillment with faith. The believer can intellectually employ the Word and Personal Factors, but faith ultimately determines the final outcome. It is impossible to possess the tangible results of the intangible desire until faith is employed (see Concept vs. Reality). However, with spiritual insight the believer can begin to accommodate the desire before it actually "materializes."

Jesus confirms that the Centurions request would be honored, and directs the Centurion to return home. The Centurion begins his journey home believing that there will be good news when he arrives. While he was on the way home, he received the news that His servant was healed (Matt. 8:13; Luke 7:2-10). Jesus stated to the lepers to go wash themselves, and show themselves to the priest. The lepers demonstrated their faith by proceeding as Jesus instructed. In each case and numerous others the persons began operating according to the desire of their heart's before the desire actually materializes.

The Confirmation Factor

When the believer is left to consider God's will alone, there is the potential that the believer's biases will skew the decision or choice. The believer should consult two or three other believers in regards to a potential decision, particularly when the decision is considered extremely important.

These other persons should be believers who possess the spiritual maturity necessary to assist in the process. Furthermore, they should support their views with Biblical principles. It is also advisable that these individuals not be persons who will simply agree due to their subordinate position, or agree due to a conflict of interest. Neither should the believer select someone who does not understand the concepts of faith. Clearly, the believer seeking confirmation must understand that all believers are not capable of providing valuable spiritual or practical insight.

Once the believer has evaluated the alternatives alone with two or three others, and they also agree upon the alternative, the believer can proceed with the decision.

This process of confirmation is used in determining the trust worthiness of a person's testimony or condition, and it is therefore useful in other areas (Matt. 18:16). Likewise, the agreement of two or three believers that does not violate any other Biblical principle will be honored by the Father (Matt. 18:18,19).

The Sovereignty Factor

The believer must be reminded that God is completely autonomous. That is, it may appear that nothing is operating according to His Word. The believer may be convinced that every Biblical principle has been satisfied. The believer is obedient, humble, faithful, and demonstrates every spiritual fruit conceivable. However, believers must remember that God performs according to His desire, and the believer's comprehensive needs. The believer's comprehensive needs involve the operation of all entities and conditions in the angelic and natural dimensions. Often, this is not obvious to the believer. The Spirit knows every need, socially, psychologically, physically, and [more importantly], spiritually (Matt. 6:8).

Furthermore, while He provides for us on earth, His ultimate purpose for our lives is our eternal destiny (Matt. 25:46; John 12:25). Understanding the five factors of determining God's will greatly enhances an individual's ability to make the right choice.

Life Transformation Not Behavior Modification

From the view of the Christ-based Counselor, the believer's life is renewed through spiritual birth where the process of transformation begins. Rebirth represents a transformation to a "new life" compared to proponents of behavior modification where the effort is to modify the old life. Christ-based Counseling exceeds the psycho-socio model that holds that behavior is best modified by drug or non-medicinal exercises. These pale in comparison when the comprehensive needs are considered. Even powerful medicinal therapies cannot change the counselee's environment, circumstances, or issues of the soul, and there's always the concern with side-effects. While behavior modification is noteworthy in terms of its discussion of processes, which mold the personality such as positive reinforcement, behavior modification has serious defects.

The Consummate Personality

Among many problems, psycho-socio therapies do not have a universally accepted prototype. The social environment of the United

States and most of the Western world varies on the question, "what is acceptable behavior"? The use of expletives is common place in board rooms across America. The marketing and consumption of alcoholic beverages is a multibillion dollar industry. Pornographic material is a legal, and widely accepted form of entertainment. Premarital sex is an accepted reality. Even the Church has succumbed to the changing world of behavior with homosexual pastors, polygamist and similar matters. Again, the question is "what is acceptable behavior"?

A New Creation

Another problem with behavior modification is the presumption that the "old life" can be modified. Attempting to modify the existing nature of the old life with a body of principles designed to govern behavior is as futile as placing new wine in old bottles (Matt. 9:17).

What the believer has in Jesus is a new life to live including: (1) a prototype of behavior to visualize (Matt. 5:17), (2) access to the power that will assist the believer in conforming to the prototype (John 1:12; 4:26; 16:13), (3) provisions for forgiveness of sins (Matt.9:6).

Christ-based "Preinforcement"

What the behaviorist calls positive reinforcement, the Christ-based Counselor refers to as "merited" favor. Positive reinforcement says to the human being "you do something good or acceptable, I will reward your for it, or you do something positive and positive things will happen." Notwithstanding one's condition, Christ-based Counseling begins with the premise that God has already provided a magnificent gift to the counselee. The counselee has only to receive the gift to enter the frontier of a new life, where God will provide the "opportunity" to fulfill every need and desire (Matt. 6:33; 16:19; 21:22; Mark 4:24; 11:23; John 14:13; 15:16; 16:23).

"Preinforcement Continuum"

"Preinforcement" continuum represents the fact that the initial gift or stimuli provided by God through Jesus Christ is intended as the foundation for endless provisions. In contrast to the behaviorist who only operates in the natural realm, the believer through the power of the Holy Spirit has the support of the supernatural. The counselee has the assurance that sacrificing personal preferences for Christian principles will be rewarded (Matt. 10:37-42; John 14:15,21; 15:10,11). Unlike positive reinforcement were the stimuli or reward is typically proportionate to the behavior desired, the believer's rewards immeasurably exceed any personal sacrifices (Matt. 19:29). Briefly stated, these rewards represent a continuum of the original gift (John 10:10b).

Antecedents of Pavlov's Respondent Conditioning

As the counselee experiences and interprets the results of decisions made in Christ, the counselee establishes the propensity to continue to make the faithful and obedient decisions. The net result is an individual who is not simply living an old life with new habits. The outcome is a transformed organism, who is being constantly conformed to the image of Jesus Christ (Matt. 10:24,25; Luke 6:40 John 3:3;10:10; Rom. 8:29).

Beyond Heredity and Environment

The Christ-based Counselor cannot avoid the realities of the impact of heredity and environment on the counselee. The counselor has the responsibility to discover as much about both of these factors as possible. In practical terms heredity and environment are defined as follows:

Hereditary factors include biological traits which affect all aspects of the human anatomy, particularly those which influence decisions. A review of parents, grandparents, siblings and other relatives would be appropriate. Issues such as health, personal habits, and any other hereditary related factors assist in an evaluation of one's heredity.

Environmental factors include all of the experiences, living conditions, and interaction with one's environment. The counselor must attempt to discover as much as possible about these factors and their relationship to the counselee.

The Christ-based Counselor recognizes that the potential to resolve a counselee's problem is not confined to the limitations imposed by heredity or environmental factors. Possessing an understanding that parents have a "genetic" influence on their children, the disciples asked Jesus about the man blind from his childhood (John 9:2), "Master, who did sin, this man, or his parents, that he was born blind?" Perhaps the disciples never studied physiology or biogenetics, but they had a grasp of the realities of heredity. There is a sense that their question actually inferred a specific sin or a life of sin.

Heredity (Nature)

Nevertheless, the disciples recognized the patrimonial aspect of sin. Both sin and humanity combine to propagate man's condition to each generation including all the results of the original sin (i.e., sickness, disease, etc.). A mainstay of the Christ-based Counselor's approach is derived from the answer Jesus gives His disciples in regards to their presumption. "Neither, 'Jesus answered.' But to demonstrate the power of God." Jesus does not refute the validity of their presupposition. However, the disciples' focus was misdirected. The most important concern was not how the man's condition was inherited.

Merely diagnosing and labeling a symptom with psychobabble does nothing to resolve the issue. Typically, symptoms are obvious or else the counselee would not seek assistance. The question is, HOW CAN THE MAN'S CONDITION BE REMEDIED?

The Christ-based Counselor must not languish in the far reaches of investigative analysis. The Christ-based Counselor must understand the hereditary concerns, but resist the temptation to continually rehash them with the counselee. After conducting discovery of the counselee's background, develop techniques or counseling policy determined to focus on helping the person to do the will of the Father (i.e., exhibit the behavior, attitude, or condition consistent with principles in the Christian faith). Do not allow the counselee to remain in the past (Matt. 8:22). Regardless of the depth of despair suggested by the counselee's heredity, his or her condition is an opportunity "that the works of God might be shown" in the counselee.

Environment (Nurture)

Environmental factors were also alluded to in the Gospels. How often was issue taken with the thought that Jesus was merely a carpenter's son? Here, Jesus was constantly reminded that His destiny was limited by the social status of His parents. The religious leaders were also astonished by His association with the dregs of society (i.e., drunkards, tax collectors, promiscuous types, etc.). Perhaps the most classic reference to the influence of environment was made in reference to Jesus, "Can there anything good come from Nazareth (John 1:46)." The fact that Jesus was actually born in Bethlehem is not the issue. The salient point is that Nathaniel recognized the effect a person's environment can have on an individual's life. Obviously from Nathaniel's statement, the environment of Nazareth produced notorious misfits and criminal types. As with the hereditary issues, the environmental factors must be understood to the degree possible. However, a counselee's gloomy environmental conditions must not be accepted as an occasion to surrender. In complete awe of Jesus' omniscience, Nathaniel answers his own question in regards to Nazareth when he says to Jesus, "Rabbi, thou art the Son of God; thou art the King of Israel" (John 1:49). The Christ-based Counselor must recognize that success can emerge from an environmental disaster.

Hard Core Cases

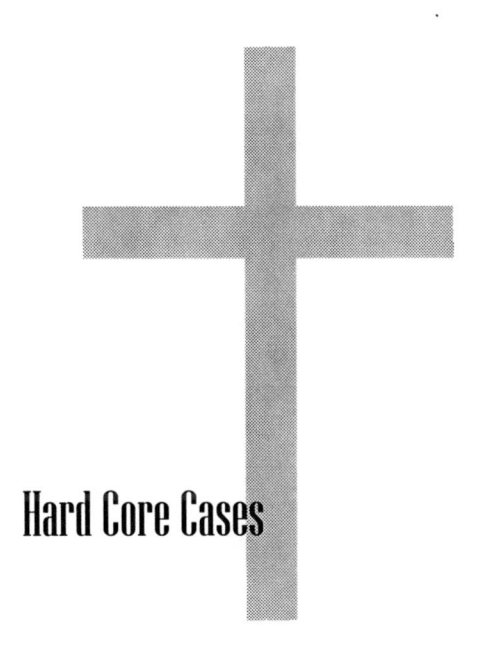

Is Christ-based Counseling Limited? A number of issues and examples are offered by "Christian" psychology professionals as conditions exceeding the bounds of Christ-based Counselors. An example of these "Hard Core" cases are as follows:

> Homosexuality
> Anorexia, Bulimia
> Cross Dressers
> Victims of Incest and Molestation
> Other extreme forms of behavioral deviance

Clearly, these are cases that should be identified as red flags for any counselor, secular or Christ-based.

These cases should not be "typical" for the Christ-based Counselors whose counseling is limited to persons who are members of the Christian faith. Nevertheless, these problems are evident within the body of Christ.

Those Christian and secular professionals who do not believe that Christ-based Counseling is an acceptable approach to the non-organic

Hard Core cases are misguided.

Beyond Simple Exhortations

The Hard-core cases definitely exceed the intentions of a simple exhortation to righteous living presented in a Biblical quotation or a Bible study. Anyone with such an approach has seriously underestimated the depth of these illnesses.

However devoid of any organic problems, these cases do not require an exhaustive psychological examination of the counselee's psycho-social framework, and an accompanying battery of therapies.

Understanding Humanity from a Christ-based Construct

Jesus provides an extraordinary view of the human organism, which will be helpful at this point:

"Quadmetric" View of Man

There are a number of different views of what constitutes the human organism. Some believe that man is a dichotomy. That is, man is body and soul. Some hold a position that man is tripartite. Man is body, soul, and spirit. There is Biblical support for both of these. However, I believe the most definitive finding about man was revealed by Jesus. Jesus was engaged in a conversation when a religious man asked about the most important commandment. Jesus' reply helps us understand the inner workings of mankind:

And thou shalt love the Lord thy God with all thy heart, and with all thy soul, and with all thy mind, and with all thy strength: this is the first commandment
(Mark 12:30, KJV).

Note, there are four distinct characteristics of mankind which are involved in demonstrating love toward God. These four functions within man must demonstrate a certain standard. Love is the standard or metric. This is the origin of the term, "quadmetric" view. Jesus' first instruction is to love God with the heart. Obviously, the physical heart is not where love can reside. Jesus means to love God with our spirit. This spirit, which Jesus references is different than the Holy Spirit. Jesus likely means that a person's disposition, demeanor, or behavior pattern should represent a love and reverence for God. While it exceeds the scope of this book, there is no doubt that one's spirit is at the core of a persons disposition. Secondly, Jesus speaks of loving God with all of one's soul. The soul is the seat of emotions. The person who loves God does so with an emotional response that is consistent with the truths in God's Word. Thirdly, loving God with the mind involves the cognitive process. This is where thinking occurs. Thinking is based on God's Word as opposed to the world's system or logic. Finally, loving God with all of one's strength. This appears to be physical, but is also all encompassing. Loving with all of one's strength involves what the believer does, where the believer goes, how the believer acts and more.

Once the religious leader repeated and affirmed what Jesus stated, verse 34 discloses the following:

And when Jesus saw that he answered discreetly, he said unto him, Thou art not far from the kingdom of God. And no man after that durst ask him any question (Mark 12:33, KJV).

While the specific topic of discussion involved the most important commandment, we are able to deduce from the statement the four parts of mankind. The text further shows that the man answered discreetly. This an affirmation of the detailed parts of man as well as the principal commandment.

As shown above the heart can also be rendered behavior pattern. Treasures, which offer great satisfaction are the ones that dominate the behavior.

Jesus instructed his followers about an inherent quality of human beings. People are self-gratification oriented (Matt. 10:39; 16:25). The instruments or objects of self-gratification can be identified as treasures. These treasures can exist in any form including material possessions, objects, lifestyles, habits, social status, position, emotional behavior, relationships, etc. (Matt. 19:16-22).

All of a person's energies are directed toward these treasures, which in-turn fulfills one's drive for self-gratification. Ironically, an individual may even understand or be aware of the depravity and/or danger of his or her condition. Nevertheless, the behavior does not cease to provide some degree of satisfaction (i.e., comfort, defense, notoriety, e.g.).

A Condition of the Heart

These extremely desperate situations can only be understood in the same context as someone who is suffering from congestive heart failure. The Christ-based Counseling model refers to these as Hard-Core conditions. This is when a person's life is completely dominated by this condition, and the activities will literally lead to death.

As stated earlier the behavior, act, event, or objects can be identified as treasures, which offer some degree of gratification. However, these treasures are merely manifestations of the counselee's spiritual condition.

Jesus, who already possesses a complete analysis of the Hard Core condition, provides the remedy so that the Christ-based specialist can move directly to the "heart" of the matter. He states, "where your treasures are there will your heart be also (Matthew 6:21)." Since the human organism is self-gratification oriented, those treasures offering the greatest satisfaction dominate the human mind and behavior.

These "treasures" are assigned an extremely high priority. In fact, these treasures become as meaningful as life itself. Therefore, the Hard-core Case counselee will not cease unhealthy behavior. The homosexual with great arrogance boasts of his sexual preference. The molester continues his acts of debauchery in spite of the criminal implications. The cross-dresser cannot refrain from his escapades with the apparel of the opposite sex. The anorectic or bulimic will not cease self-deprecating behavior. These and many others are seeking their treasures which in-turn provides a sense of self-gratification as bizarre and twisted as it may seem.

Notwithstanding why the behavior occurs (e.g., fear, harmful experience, defense mechanism, self-image, peer pressure, similar factors), God's Word in Jesus Christ provides the explanation, and His

Word provides the approach.

The "Process of Being Made Whole," and the specific CBC approach is as effective with Hard-core Counseling cases as with the cases which are more typical (marital, parental, emotional, etc.).

A Counseling Technique

Several steps should be taken to assist the counselee in overcoming Hard-core or any other problems:

1. The counselee needs an explanation of the depth of his or her condition as defined in this chapter.
2. The counselee must recognize that some degree of gratification is being experienced by his or her behavior.
3. The counselee must re-examine the depth of his or her relationship to living as a believer.
4. Christian virtues must replace the counselee's treasures. The counselee must view life from God's perspective, particularly in regards to priorities. However, this will not occur until the counselee "sacrifices" his or her own treasures for heavenly ones (Matt. 9:21-22).
5. The counselee needs a long term support group with regular meetings.
6. A timeline must be monitored to highlight periods when the hard core behavior is repeated.
7. As the counselee surpasses milestones or goals, some form of recognition should be acknowledged.
8. Cautiously, and with the agreement of the counselee, a select number of persons (2 or 3) should be made aware of the counselee's problem. These persons must be extremely trustworthy individuals who love and care for the counselee. These individuals must not violate the confidentiality of the counselee. This approach provides an additional guard for the counselee when he or she is aware that there are others who know of the problems. The temptation is more enticing when the counselee is under the impression that the unwanted behavior will not be detected. Again this technique should only be considered in the most extreme cases where the counselee desires maximum support (Matt. 18:15-16; John 8:32-36).

Monitoring Progress of the Hard Core Case

If the counselee does not experience any detectable progress over a period of time (e.g., one year), then the counselor must examine the counselee's confession of faith. Is the counselee truly "born-again"?

If the counselee is born again (John 3:7), and the counselee has allowed God's Word to take root in his or her heart (Matt. 13:23), and the counselee confesses the depravity of his or her acts (John 8:10-11; Luke 7:37-38, 47-48, 50), it is impossible for the counselee to remain in the same condition with the same level of sin-filled activity. There is not one Biblical principle to support the coexistence of long-term depravity (i.e., sin) and the spiritually born-again believer.

The Unparalleled Sufficiency of Christ-based Counseling

Christ-based Counseling is only limited to the sphere of man's ability to believe God. Even the organic problems are within God's ability. However, with great caution the believer recognizes the potential problems related to cases relative to organic conditions. Certainly if a medical physician has the remedy, the counselor is advised to recommend the counselee to the appropriate physician or medical advisor. Nevertheless, Christ-based Counseling is not limited.

Again, no therapy has been more successful in healing the conditions of mankind than the individual who surrenders to a Christ-based approach. The words of John give testimony to the incredible record of the Master counselor when he (i.e., John) states "And there are also many other things which Jesus did, which if they were written in detail, I suppose that even the world itself would not contain the books which were written." Freudians, Skinnerians, Rogerians, Adlerians, Jungians, Ellisonians, et al., combined cannot boast of the success in healing the ills of man as those who operate through Christ-Jesus.

Endnotes

1. Charles Erdman, The Gospel of Matthew (Philadelphia: The Westminster Press, 1975), p. 146
2. Howard Clark Kee, The Interpreter's One Volume Commentary (Nashville: Abingdon Press, 1971), p. 628
3. Charles F. Pfeiffer & Everett F. Harrison (ed.), The Wycliffe Bible Commentary (Chicago: Moody Press, 1962), p. 958
4. Matthew Henry, Matthew Henry's Commentary on the Whole Bible, 6 vols. (New York: Fleming H. Revell Co., n.d.), V:225ff.

Christ-based Counseling (CBC)
The Process of Being Made Whole

The core of Christ-based Counseling (CBC) is the Process of Being Made Whole. This Process includes six constituents and strategic prayer for forty-five days. Regardless of the issue, it is important for the counselee to understand these factors.

The Counselee Must Be Born-Again (John 3:3-8): The foundation of Christ-based Counseling's effectiveness is in the faith dimension. Therefore, only persons who are believers can avail themselves to the therapeutic or healing process in Christ-based Counseling. Persons who do not know the Lord, but desire CBC must be evangelized first. Nevertheless, Jesus' discussion with Nicodemus in the referenced text makes the point clear. The counselee must be born again.

The Counselee Must Be Presented Balanced Biblical Insights (Matt. 4:5-7): God's Word, rightly divided is the therapy for right thinking. However, as shown in the referenced text, God's Word must be balanced and not some misapplied presentation of God's Word. This can be seen in the Devil's inappropriate use of Psalms 91. Christ-based Counseling relies on the appropriate use of God's Word, and understands the overarching principles of God's Word.

The Counselee Must Possess the Degree of Faith Needed (Mark 4:24): Beyond possessing faith unto salvation, counselees must believe that God will intervene in their personal circumstances. The referenced verse is preceded by verses 13-20 where Jesus explains the different types of hearers of God's Word: Wayside, Stony, Thorns & Thistles, and Good Ground. Each of these persons represents how "hearers" embrace God's Word. Regardless of the circumstances, Good Ground hearers <u>believe</u>. They believe that God "is" operating in their personal situation.

The Counselee Must Be Committed (Luke 21:1-4): Counselees must be thoroughly invested in the Process. The woman in the example gave "all" that she had. What a difference she represents compared to the typical person in our culture. Often people do not desire to make the investment of time and personal sacrifice. This Process requires complete commitment by the counselee as the woman shown in the referenced text.

The Counselee Must Do The Practical (Mark 8:1-3): Depending on the issue, counselees must do the practical or physical things. As shown in the referenced text, Jesus recognizes the need to feed the multitude, or they would faint. The practical matters must be satisfied, and these are usually understood. As an example, a person seeking a job must seek employment opportunities, and submit applications where applicable.

The Counselee Must Stay In The Process (John 15:3-9): Persons who encounter any issue must be willing to invest time in counseling, prayer, study, and application of God's Word. It is popular to look for the immediate answer and quick solution. However, the essence of a problem is that the answer may not result in an immediate resolution. Therefore, counselees must stay in the counseling process as scheduled. Also, they must be engaged in the greater fellowship of believers, and on-going development in Christ.

Forty-Five Days of Prayer

Important to the counseling process is the additional therapeutic dimension of strategic prayer. As opposed to generalized prayer, the term strategic is used to denote the specific focus of prayer. Remember, Christ-based Counseling works with both dimensions (i.e., the natural and spiritual). The Lord has empowered believers to impact the spiritual dimension.

Why Forty-five Days? As mentioned in the sixth constituent of the Process of Being Made Whole, issues faced by most counselees represent problems that will not be resolved in a short timeframe. Additionally, many believers do not have a daily and concentrated prayer regimen.

Most important life changes require a transition, which usually involves the combination of an established timeframe and a different behavioral pattern, focus, or practice.

Biblically, the number forty is used so often it is more than a mere coincident. Other significant numbers, which most of us hear about are three and seven. There are others not mentioned as significantly.

One must be cautious about the use of numbers. There is always the danger that one may be overcome by superstition and mysticism involving numbers. Praying for forty-five days has nothing to do with any kind of superstition.

Biblically, [after sin] it appears that it requires a timeframe of about forty earth days or years for the operation of angels to complete an assignment. The term, "earth days" are used for our (i.e., human) benefit. Angels are the purveyors of God's will. That is, they are the workers at God's command who cause results in the material universe. God uses the angels to create, change, or allow our circumstances. They work in the angelic dimension, but their results are manifested in the physical dimension. Clearly, God has connected our prayers to their operation. There are more than 250 references to angels in the Bible.

Since angels are not limited by time or space, they merely refer to days for our benefit (e.g., Dan. 10:13). Therefore, the events in Scripture involving "forty" often refer to the completion of a phase, process, or administration. If this is true, the principle should be witnessed at least three times in Scripture (Deuteronomy 17:6; Matthew 18:16). Examples are provided as follows:

Genesis 7:12: It rained forty days and forty nights (i.e., the Flood) before the renewal of the earth.

Numbers 13:25: Moses commissioned spies to assess the land for forty days. They returned before making their final decision concerning the Promised Land. When they were found to be unfaithful, they wandered for forty years.

Deuteronomy 10:10: Both times the tablets of the Ten Commandments required forty days to complete before being presented to the Hebrews.

I Kings 19:5-8: Prompted by two angels to eat, afterwards, Elijah fasts for forty days and nights before journeying to Mt. Horeb. There, he received transition instructions.

Ezekiel 4:6: God instructed the prophet to lie on his side for forty days as an object lesson to Judah representing the years of Judah's iniquity.

Daniel 10:13, 20: Bewildered about a vision, Daniel prays for understanding. The angel reveals that it took him twenty-one days to arrive, but the angel's mission was not concluded. He had to return and continue his battle with the prince of Persia--at least another 21 days.

Jonah 3:4: The prophet warned Nineveh that it had forty days before being overthrown. They repented and averted their doom.

The Old Testament is where the precedent is found for the significance of a timeframe covering at least forty days. More importantly, there are two extraordinary events in the life of Jesus involving forty-day periods. **First**, the gospels (Matthew 4:2; Mark 1:3; Luke 4:2) record Jesus' wilderness journey before initiating His earthly ministry. This period launching His earthly ministry was forty days and forty nights. Angels were on the scene ministering to Him (Matt. 4:11; Mark 1:13). **Secondly**, as an irrefutable demonstration of His resurrection, Jesus appeared and ministered for a period of forty days (Acts 1:3). Again, angels were on the scene as He departed earth (Acts 1:10-11).

It is noteworthy here that one of the important characteristics Jesus taught about prayer was persistency (Luke 11:5-8; Luke 18:1-8). Luke 18:1 provides the specific purpose for the instructions on prayer. Pointedly, He instructed that we must not <u>loose heart</u> (KJV) or <u>give up</u> (NIV). The Apostle Paul used terms such as "pray without ceasing" and "always praying" (Eph. 6:18; Col. 1:3; I Th. 5:17).

Recall the case where a boy was psychotic (Matt. 17:14-21), and the disciples could not cure him. Jesus rebuked the demon in the boy, and he was cured. The disciples wanted to know why they could not cure the boy. Jesus identified the problem: Their lack of faith demonstrated by the absence of prayer and fasting. Persistency in prayer is the evidence of faithfulness. Therefore, Jesus did not mean they did not pray at the moment of need. He meant, "This could only be done by persons with a discipline of prayer and fasting." The most challenging issues in life require a <u>process</u> of faith demonstrated by persistent prayer disciplines (i.e., prayer and fasting). Disciples/persons with these virtues need only to strategically focus on a specific need. Like Jesus, their angels are "on-the-ready" awaiting marching orders from the Lord (Matt. 18:10; 26:51-53). **NOTE:** Believers must not worship, or pray to angels.

Clearly, Jesus knew the reality of what happens in the angelic dimension when believers pray. The angels are on the move, but they are opposed. God has connected their success to our faith or persistence. Jesus says, "don't loose heart." We must keep praying on a specific issue.

Finally, Ephesians 6:10-20 discusses the opposition to believers' walk in Christ. Paul makes it clear that the overwhelming objective must be to defeat demonic operations in the angelic dimension. Once this is accomplished, the way is cleared for "results" in the physical or material dimension. Please notice that the weaponry is spiritual. The Christ-based Counseling focus is verses 16-18. These verses highlight faith, the Spirit or Word of God, and prayer as the primary weapons. Paul adds, "… and watching with all perseverance …" No doubt, God can resolve a matter in a day. However, the Biblical evidence is convincing that a process is required for matters requiring spiritual intervention.

Finally, the term, "forty years" is also noteworthy. "Forty years" is used more often than "forty days." Consider that with God and the angels, there is no difference between forty-days, and forty-years (Psalms 90:4; 2 Peter 3:8). When believers pray in a range of forty days--in God's will, they will see a discernable change. Remember, this affirms a process or practice in the angelic dimension. The issue may not be resolved, but there will be change. In addition, a person will be closer to the Lord's answer. Obviously, some matters of prayer will be with us a lifetime. Others are not long at all.

Test it! If you have an issue, follow the six-steps, and pray forty-five days. See if there is an affirmative "change." Remember, the number, "forty" is not magical. One is to keep praying until the mission is complete.

Who is the origin of the additional five days? As Paul would say, "this is not the Lord's command, but mine and I believe it is worthy. An additional five days cannot hurt." sbd

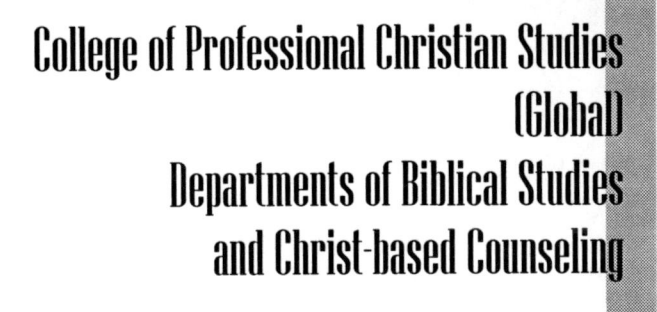

College of Professional Christian Studies (Global)
Departments of Biblical Studies and Christ-based Counseling

COURSE: Process of Being Made Whole (6 constituents and 45 days of prayer)

Practicum Requirement:

Course Literature: CBC Study and Bible

Pre-requisites (if any):

Understanding the Course Design

Students use the literature to respond to questions. Questions are in chronological order throughout the course. Questions preceded with bracket statements require Biblical, spiritual, or counseling insight and these questions test the student's ability to deduce, assimilate, and otherwise process a number of factors to answer the questions.

Completion requirements are as follows:

Sections: The course is divided into several sections of approximately 50 questions each. It is not necessary to complete all sections in one setting. However, you must complete a section before submitting your work. DO NOT submit a section that is partially complete.

1. What is the core of Christ-based Counseling?

2. How many constituents comprise the process?

3. What is the first step in the Process of Being Made Whole?

4. Where is the foundation of Christ-based Counseling's effectiveness?

5. Who are the only persons who can avail themselves to CBC?

6. What must persons do first, who do not know the Lord?

7. According to Jesus, what is necessary for any person who desires a therapy where faith is involved?

8. What is the second step in the Process of Being Made Whole?

9. What is the therapy for right thinking?

10. Read the referenced text (Matt. 4:5-7).

11. Satan wants Jesus to prove that He (Jesus) is the son of God. What does Satan use as the "authority" to convince Jesus that his (Satan's) request is legitimate? (Hint: Satan makes a reference to it in verse 6,"for it ...")

12. What does Jesus use as His "authority" responding to Satan's request?

13. What verse in Scripture does Satan attempt to misuse?

14. What does Christ-based Counseling rely on?

15. What is the third step in the Process that counselees must possess?

16. What must counselees believe in the third step?

17. Name the four different types of hearers?

18. Read Mark 4:13-20, which of the hearers has God's Word snatched before it can take root in the heart?

19. Which of the hearers receives God's word, but "gives-up" upon experiencing difficulties as the result of obeying God's Word?

20. What are the characteristics of the Thorns & Thistles hearer?

21. Who <u>believes</u> in spite of the circumstances?

22. According to this step, the more a person believes and applies God's Word, the more...? (Complete the sentence/thinking)

23. Write the fourth step.

24. How much did the widow in the text give in life's value? (Hint: not monetary value)

25. What is ironic about our culture concerning lifestyle change?

26. What does the Process require?

27. What is the fifth step in the Process?

28. Read Mark 8:1-3. How long were the people with Jesus?

29. What physical necessity did Jesus recognize?

30. What is used as an example of completing a practical matter?

31. What is the final step in the Process?

32. Read John 15:3-9. What verb does Jesus repeat several times during the reading?

33. What will counselees be willing to do?

34. What makes most issues problematical?

35. Name two functions counselees must observe.

36. What additional therapeutic dimension is extremely important?

37. Are most problems resolved in a short timeframe?

38. Do many believers have a daily and concentrated prayer regimen?

39. What do most life changes require?

40. Name two factors necessary to reach a lifestyle change.

41. What number is used so often in the Bible that it is clearly more than a coincident?

42. What other numbers are seen often in the Bible?

43. What must believers be cautious about concerning numbers?

44. After sin, what is apparent concerning the timeframe of about forty days?

45. What is meant by the term, "Angels are purveyors of God's will?"

Course ▪ 67

46. What specifically do angels accomplish?

47. Where do angels work?

48. What has God connected to their operation?

49. How many references to angels are in the Bible?

50. Why do angels refer to days in the Bible (e.g., Dan. 10:13)?

51. Events in the Bible involving "forty" refer to the completion of a _____, _____, or _____. (Fill in blanks)

52. If the principle concerning "forty" is true, how many times should it be shown in the Bible?

53. What happens in Genesis 7:12?

54. What happens in Numbers 13:25?

55. What happens in Deuteronomy 10:10?

56. What happens in I Kings 19:5-8?

57. What was the prophet instructed to do in Ezekiel 4:6?

58. How many days did it take the angel to arrive upon Daniel's request?

59. Was the angel's mission over when He arrived to Daniel?

60. How long do you think it would take for the angel to complete the mission? Why?

61. How long did Nineveh have to repent in Jonah 3:4?

62. Are there more than two or three references to the use of forty days in the Bible? (Shown in the questions above)

63. Where is the precedent found for the principle concerning forty days?

64. More importantly, give two examples in the New Testament where the forty-day principle is evident.

65. Who was on the scene in both cases?

66. What is one of the most important characteristics of prayer in Luke 11:5-8; and Luke18:1-8?

67. In Luke 11:5-8, what does the man desire from his neighbor?

68. Was his original request provided?

69. Given his neighbor's original response, how did the man respond?

70. Recall, what is Jesus' topic in Luke 11:5-8?

71. What is the primary characteristic Jesus teaches about prayer in verses 5-8?

72. Who are the two characters in Luke 18:1-8?

73. Concerning prayer, what is Jesus' specific objective for believers in verse 1?

74. How was the widow's initial request received by the judge?

75. What type of character did the judge possess?

76. How did the widow respond to the judge's initial response to her request?

77. Eventually, how does the judge respond to the widow's request?

78. What is the primary characteristic Jesus is teaching us by the parable of the woman before the unjust judge?

79. What two terms does Paul use concerning prayer?

80. Read Matthew 17:14-21. Who was ill?

81. What were the symptoms of the boy's illness?

82. Who tried to cure the boy?

83. Why were they unsuccessful?

84. Explain what Jesus meant by His explanation for the disciples inability to cure the boy?

85. What do the most challenging issues in life require?

86. What must be demonstrated, persistently?

87. When believers have a consistent prayer discipline, who is waiting for marching orders from the Lord?

88. Believers must not worship or pray to what beings?

89. What did Jesus know concerning the angelic dimension?

90. Angelic success is often connected to our _____ (fill in space).

91. Read Ephesians 6:10-20. What does Paul make clear?

92. Once the "overwhelming objective" is accomplished, what is cleared?

93. What type of weaponry does Paul address?

94. What are the focal verses in Ephesians Chapter 6 for PBMW?

95. What do verses 16-18 highlight?

96. What else does Paul add?

97. What can God do in a single day?

98. What is required for most matters requiring spiritual intervention?

99. What other term is also noteworthy? Concerning God and angels is there any difference between the two?

100. When believers pray in a range of forty days, what will they experience?

101. Will issues always be resolved in forty days? Explain. Where does the additional five days come from?

Christ-based Counseling (CBC)

Illustrated

Christ-based Counseling Preparation and Distinction

Christ-based Counseling Preparation

Persons who are reading this book are seeking wholeness for one's self or others. There are three functional investments counselees or other participants must make in Christ-based Counseling (CBC) exercises. The participant must:

- ✓ READ
- ✓ RESPOND
- ✓ REITERATE

This means the counselee reads the information, answers each question, and discusses or shares the answers with another person. The questions are divided into blocks of fifty questions each session. The participant can be any person interested in the process (e.g., minister, counselor, friend, relative, etc.).

Whether it is used with or without a Christ-based Counselor, the most effective use of the Christ-based Counseling approach is to begin with the Process of Being Made Whole. I strongly recommend that you complete the Process of Being Made Whole (PBMW) as a prerequisite to the specific counseling needed.

The Process of Being Made Whole, and accompanying course is on the internet at Christbasedcounseling.org. Simply click-on the link or door for the School of Counseling and Certification, and scroll down to The Process of Being Made Whole link. Print out the on-line guide. Use the guide to answer the questions in the on-line course. This on-line course link is the next link beneath the Process of Being Made Whole link.

The Process of Being Made Whole and questions are also included in this book for your convenience. Both the guide and questions are a mirror image of the web versions. If you have completed the Process of Being Made Whole previously, and you have mastered all seven constituents, you may skip the Process of Being Made Whole.

Christ-based Counseling's Distinction

I have counseled literally hundreds of couples and individuals. And unlike the psychological and medical professions, I assure counselees there will be positive change in forty-five days. Persons who meticulously follow each step and who stay-the-course over time may not resolve the issues they face in forty-five days, but there will be change. And they will establish significant progress toward the wholeness they seek. This is because the principles in Christ-based Counseling operate in the angelic realm where the most effective powers and authorities operate to change the physical realm.

Christ-based Counseling is also distinguished from Christian counseling or Christian psychology where the basis is often psychotherapy under the guise of sprinkled scripture text. Christ-based Counseling is based on a sound Scriptural system where the whole approach is thoroughly Biblical.

Finally, this is not a novel, motivational guide, or academic text. This approach is a spiritually empowered process with principles to be observed for the remainder of your life. Typically, the behavior and habits we desire to overcome have been with us for years. Therefore, it may be necessary to review the Christ-based Counseling principles numerous times.

Marriage, Divorce, and the Believer

This document is for clergy, counselors, and persons who know someone who needs balanced biblical answers, and practical emotional help. The document gives Biblical illustrations of our emotions, and strategies to assist the counselor and counselee in marital crisis.

The Divorce Phenomena

No trend in American family life since World War II has received more attention or caused more concern than the rising rate of divorce. The divorce rate, however, has been rising since at least the middle of the nineteenth century. It is true that the rise in annual divorce rates in the 1960s and 1970s is much steeper and more sustained than any increase in the past century [1].

By the mid-1970s for the first time in our nation's history, more marriages ended every year in divorce than in death [2]. One of the most important effects of the rise in divorce is the number of parents whose marriages are dissolved while their children are still at home. According to 1973 data analyzed by Larry Bumpass and Ronald R. Rindfuss, seventeen percent of children born between 1968 and 1970 experienced a disrupted family by age five, as against only eleven percent of children born between 1956 and 1958 [3]. The prediction in the early 1970s was that one-third of all white children and three-fifths of all black children born between 1970 and 1973 would experience family disruption by age sixteen if the rates of 1973 hold [4].

Most of these disruptions result, at least temporarily in a one-parent family consisting of a mother and her children. Typically, mothers keep custody of their children in most instances.

During 1979, 75% of the children living in a one-parent home lived with their mother. Only seven percent lived with their fathers[5]. Earlier in the century it was common for divorced parents to send their children to live with relatives or for divorced mothers to take their children and move in with relatives.

Today, however, most currently divorced mothers live alone with their children. Much has been written about the social and economic situation of parents and children in one-parent families. This will be discussed in a later chapter, Times of Struggle Revisited.

In the face of overwhelming statistical evidence, it is understandable why divorce has become such an overwhelming reality in the Christian community. Nevertheless, marriages with believing spouses continue to persevere better than marriages with non-believing spouses (i.e., 45.6 general public[1] vs. 35% born-again[2]). Since the general public information includes born-again believers, the testimony of being born-again is even more significant. Clearly, the actual general public statistics excluding born-again believers exceeds 50%. This is a different view and finding. It is being highly publicized that born-again believers' divorce rate is the same as the general public[3]. Contrariwise, born-again couples continue to operate as a major success factor when compared to the general population. One of the major objectives of this document is to continue the battle against troubled Christian marriages.

The Formative Years

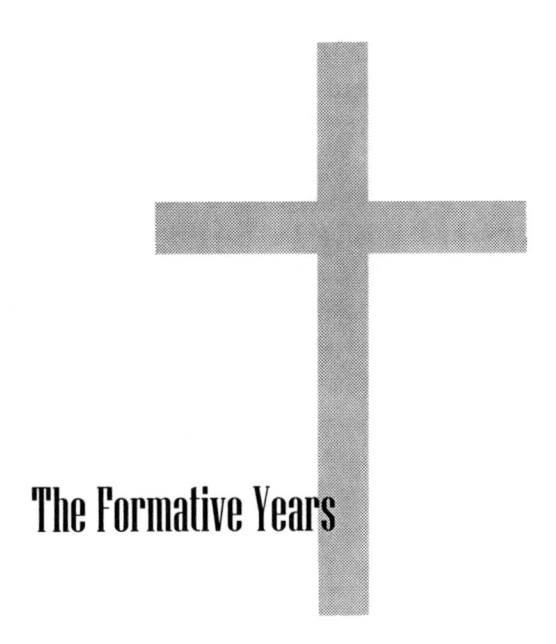

What are the dynamics involved when two people, a man and woman decide they will enter into a relationship requiring the greatest commitment to another human being. It is interesting to note that we do not make such a vow to any other human being "till death, do we part." However, before the traditional vow is examined along with its spiritual implications, an evaluation of the beginnings of the marital commitment is in order.

The Days of Wine and Roses

Here is the typical boy meets girl (or visa versa). Don meets Marie and becomes interested in her. There is something about Marie that appeals to Don. Perhaps it is her smile, or maybe her charm.

Nevertheless, Don is hooked. During the course of time and through subsequent encounters Don makes his interest known. Perhaps Marie was not aware. Or maybe she played the part of the disinterested female, while in reality she cannot wait for him to make his move. Fortunately, they both have mutual admiration for each other, and they begin dating. Don sends Marie flowers, cards and candy. They also go on dates to the movie, fair, and other social and recreational activities. They spend time on the phone in long conversations. They discover more about each other with each passing day.

If Don or Marie leaves town for a short time, they both wonder how they actually existed before they met each other. Don and Marie are hopelessly in love. It is apparent to both of them that they were created for each other. Never before have two people ever been so compatible, so loving and reciprocal in their understanding of each other's strengths and weaknesses. This was a relationship made in heaven. Don asks Marie to marry him. And they both live happily ever after, or do they?

Evaluating the Beginnings

Using the example of Don and Marie the following "Model of Involvement" demonstrates key elements of the premarital experience.

```
MODEL OF INVOLVEMENT

Initial Recognition
Male Admiration
Subsequent Encounters
Mutual Interest
Tokens-Mementos-Keepsakes
Greater Social Involvement
Emotional Involvement
Social and Emotional Dependency
Marital Commitment
```

Fig. 1. Model of Involvement

While this is not an attempt to infer that every experience is precisely as demonstrated by the model, it serves as a general account of the process in question. The various aspects of the model may differ in sequence or concept, but usually the elements cited will be evident. Nevertheless, each event in the process is explained as follows:

Initial Recognition

It cannot be refuted that somewhere the two individuals meet. It may be at school, job, internet, church, a social gathering or any other place where males and females have a mutual experience. Whether through a friend, relative, or their own initiative the two lives intersect.

Male Admiration

Since it is obvious that the roles could be reversed with the woman (Marie) initiating the premarital activities, this section is identified as Male Admiration to maintain the consistency of the anecdote (i.e., Don and Marie) and the Model. The question is, what is it that Don admires about Marie? It could be any characteristic or combination thereof that she possesses. It primarily depends on what Don perceives as characteristics or features important to him. Don's evaluative criteria and the stages of its development can be as complex as life itself, involving his personal experiences, social and economic status, religious beliefs, political interest, etc.

Nevertheless, to answer the question is to understand what initiated the relationship in the first place.

Subsequent Encounters

Naturally, when a man is interested in a woman, he will find a way to see her though she may not be aware of his interest. And since they met at a place or through a common medium, it is only fitting that they would continue to see each other. If this is not the case, the interested party (i.e., Don) does what is necessary to ensure that he does see her if only momentarily.

Mutual Interest

Eventually, Don must inform Marie of his interest. He must convey to her that his interest is beyond a simple casual admiration. This of course may not be orally communicated. The way he communicates his intentions will depend on his personal experiences.

If Marie is interested she will accept his advances and begin to demonstrate mutual interest.

Tokens, Mementos and Keepsakes

If it has not already started, an assortment of gifts and surprises mark the relationship as something special. Flowers, cards, trinkets, pictures, necklaces, chains, rings and any number of other items demonstrate the mutual interest and gratitude.

Greater Social Involvement

The two date each other at an increasing rate. They introduce each other to family and friends. Persons who make up their environment realize the depth of their relationship. Practically all of their free time is shared with each other.

Emotional Involvement

The two become so involved with each other that one can feel or trigger an emotional response in the other. A difficult day for Don becomes an issue for Marie. A depressing day for Marie affects Don. They mutually experience the failures, disappointments, frustrations and other emotional responses of daily living. This is even more apparent when there is a misunderstanding. One of the two or perhaps both are hurt. There may be harsh words or even a period of separation. However, a combination of the passing of time and the growing dependency usually provides the impetus for reconciliation.

Social and Emotional Dependency

Depending on the scope of the involvement from a social standpoint and an emotional standpoint, eventually the couple develop a mutual dependency. And the dependency is particularly evident if the two have become sexually involved. Although premarital sex is not a part of the Model, it certainly has overwhelming implications when it becomes a part of the premarital activity. However, it does not nullify the premise of the Model. In fact, it would reinforce the model, particularly the social and emotional dependency element. This is discussed at length in Sex, Sexuality, and the Believer.

The Marital Proposal

Based on the obvious, the couple decide that marriage is a natural result of such an overwhelming social, emotional, and personal response. They make the necessary arrangements and become lawfully wedded.

Times of Struggle

"Man born of woman is of few days and full of trouble (Job 14:1 NIV)." Difficult periods in an individual's life is not an exception, it is the rule. When two people become a union each person has a multiplicity of expectations. Most of these expectations are positive and ingratiating ideas of what he or she perceives as the direction of the relationship. When either party encounters an obstacle, which limits the ability to reach or attain such expectations the natural result is frustration. An expectation does not have to be in the form of some grand childhood idea such as the size of the family, the type of home, or other similar aspirations. The marital relationship is so dependent on communications, understanding, and other relational characteristics that even the slightest personality trait can be the source of a major problem.

An excellent example of this is a couple by the name of Johnson (Larry and Lillie). Larry was a college graduate and held a management position with an established company. Lillie was also a college graduate, and also held a professional position. They became acquainted when Lillie became a member of the church where Larry was a member.

They worked on a church committee together and became mutually interested in each other. They dated and grew in their appreciation for one another. Eventually they united as man and wife.

Larry was reared in a rural setting. Lillie was an urban dweller from the days of her childhood. Larry maintained many of the characteristics that might be readily associated with a rural upbringing. And while someone born in an urban environment might possess the same traits which Larry exhibited, Lillie perceived Larry's activity as directly related to his rural background. As an example, on a hot day Larry would eat at the dining table without a shirt. Lillie was shocked by this behavior. Larry would also allow his toe nails to grow beyond an acceptable length as far as Lillie was concerned.

While Lillie's issues may not seem like a major problem to the casual observer, the fact is that they were sources of frustration and irritation to Lillie. Lillie's expectations were as important to her as any other aspiration. She expected a companion with the same mores and grooming patterns that she possessed. And when he demonstrated that he could not readily adapt her habits, it created a relational problem.

This is but one example of how delicate the marital cord can be. There are couples who would examine the Johnson's situation and long for a similar dilemma. Events or experiences, which can cause an unbearable time of struggle in a marriage can vary. However, in an effort to compile a short list of problems identified as most damaging to the marital relationship a survey was conducted. Although the survey will be evaluated in greater detail in a later chapter, results from this question are useful at this point.

CAUSES FOR MARITAL DISCORD
TABLE I

Causes	Percent
Adultery	46%
Communications problems	17%
Deception/Lying	6%
Loss of respect	6%
Christ-less relationship	6%
Immaturity/Selfishness	6%
Others (e.g., mental/physical cruelty, irresponsibility, abandonment, substance abuse)	10%

Survey Question: In your opinion what is the incident, or act that damages a marriage more than anything else?

Type of Participants: Professed Christians, primarily leaders

Number of Participants: 40

Percent of Error: This particular survey does not meet the rigid requirements for scientific accuracy. However, it does give a general view of the question asked. And there is also reason to believe that the response may not be significantly different from a survey conducted under more rigid constraints (e.g. random, proportionate to population size, sex, social status, etc.)

It is important to note, the question was not multiple choice. Each participant was allowed to "write in" an answer according to his or her own opinion. Although it is true that a marriage can encounter difficulties for many reasons, the actual contributing factors can be categorized under one of the broader causes shown in TABLE I.

Given all of the evidence, an individual entering a marital relationship must expect times or periods of struggle. It is unrealistic to enter such a relationship without recognizing that there will be difficult challenges. Nevertheless, when couples experience prolonged problems one of the inevitable alternatives is divorce. Considering divorce as an alternative is a decision, which has a tremendous effect on the divorcee and family. The question of divorce is even more significant for the Christian. The following chapters discuss a Biblical perspective of marriage and divorce. This will assist the counselor or counselee with understanding the Biblical principles concerning both.

A Study on Christian Marriage

Often, the question is asked, "what is a Christian marriage?" On the surface this appears to be a question properly stated, particularly since Jesus said, "What God has put together, let no man put asunder (Matt.19:6)." The opposite inference is, "if God did not put it together, it CAN BE put asunder." This kind of thinking is logical, but often leads to dangerous presumptions about a spouses spiritual commitment, and the intent of Matthew 19:6. When seeking alternatives to marital difficulties, the inclination for a believer with such an understanding of Matthew 19:6 is to determine whether or not the marriage is a Christian Marriage. This is often the case although they both may be confessed believers. And as further evidence, they made vows before God, and a host of Christian witnesses including a clergyman.

One evening I received a call from a Pastor's wife who realized I was involved in research on the divorce issue. She was counseling a woman on this issue, and her major concern was the woman's attempt to use Matthew 19:6 to support a cause for divorce.

Apparently, the woman had began a spiritual evaluation to determine whether her spouse was sincerely a believer. Her thinking was that if she could conclude that he truly was not a believer, the marriage was not a Christian marriage. Therefore, she could dissolve the marriage.

As far as determining whether to divorce, the Scripture does not discuss whether the marriage is a Christian Marriage. The Scripture actually offers more detail. The question is, "Is either the man or woman a believer?" If either the man or woman is a "believer," then the Biblical guidance is very specific.

I Corinthian Chapter Seven outlines the responsibly of the "believer." Beginning with verse ten it is clear, Paul the Apostle states, "it is not his charge but God's." RSV. The wife should not leave her husband, and the husband is not to divorce his wife. Here, the principle is clear. (Please see Chapter V. The Exception Clause for further discussion).

Paul continues with verse 12. The following verses represent his legal view and application of "legal principles," and not something he was necessarily told by God. This does not mean that it is of less importance. But the emphasis is different. Paul's instruction is that a believer does not divorce a spouse for non-belief. Apparently, this was an issue at Corinth. Believers considered using their religion as the reason for divorcing their non-believing spouses. Paul's emphasis here is that the believer is not to divorce the unbelieving spouse. "If he or she wants to leave then allow your spouse to leave. In such a case you are not bound" (See Deu 21:10-14 for the legal precedent Paul uses -- no doubt).

However, Paul places the legal view under Christ-based authority and provides additional guidance when the unbeliever desires to remain. Paul's reason for not divorcing an unbeliever is excellent. There is the possibility that the believer may lead the unbelieving spouse to Christ (vss. 16-17). There is a higher call to the believer to remain in the relationship for the cause of Christ. This totally belies the intent of using Matt. 19:6 as grounds for divorce. Therefore, in the context with the topic of this study, a marriage is bound by the Christian profession of either spouse, and whether or not the marriage is considered to be a Christian one is not the issue. However, there is a caveat or an exception clause that will be discussed in a later chapter.

HOW IS IT POSSIBLE TO LIVE UP TO SUCH AN OVERWHELMING RELATIONSHIP?

According to the Scriptures provided, the marriage relationship is the most intense and binding relationship known to humanity. And even marriages where both persons are confessed believers can become "unlivable." How can an individual possibly overcome such an incredible or impossible situation?

A believer's ability to remain in such a marriage depends on his or her depth of love for God's instruction (e.g., faith, prayer, obedience, dependence). We also call it, "ones spiritual commitment." Nevertheless, in the midst of convincing Scriptural support undergirding marriage, there are those who lament that it simply is not fair.

The key is in Ephesians 5:18-25. If a marriage is to survive, then these verses provide the responsibility of the husband and wife. The focus of one's love cannot simply be placed on the spouse, IT MUST BE BECAUSE OF ONE'S LOVE FOR GOD.

This love is demonstrated by the enactment of three principles. Often stated as commands, Ephesians 5 is marked by verbs in the indicative mood of Greek. Verbs like "submit" are stated as a matter of fact. A wife is a person who submits. The husband's love is in the imperative mood. Love is central to a husband's character in the same manner that God so loved the world. According to the text, a woman becomes a "New Testament" wife when she "is" one who submits. And a man becomes a "New Testament" husband when he "is" one whose principal characteristic is love. Among others, these are the principal characteristics that should be sought in a man or woman considering marriage.

Alternating "Subject" Command (vs. 21)

This command is perhaps the most overlooked in regards to the marital relationship. It states, "Be subject to one another out of reverence for Christ" (Eph. 5:21).

The word subject or submissive in some versions is translated from the Greek word hupotasso. This word has its roots in two other words hupo (under or beneath) and tasso (to arrange or assign to a certain position). Therefore, the couple alternates or shares the position of servitude depending on the needs of the relationship and capabilities of each spouse. They each place themselves in a subordinate position. Jesus demonstrated this principle. We needed salvation, and Jesus possessed the full character, qualities, and position with the Father to fulfill the need. Jesus made himself SUBJECT (hupotasso) by placing himself in a position of a servant and sacrifice. He humbled himself based upon our needs and his capabilities. And he did this in the face of rejection, criticism, and the ultimate, "death."

This principle does not eliminate the headship or ultimate family responsibility bestowed upon the man in the marital union. How couples operate concerning decisions and other issues does not terminate ultimate responsibility placed on the man.

Nevertheless, Jesus' sacrifice was not based on the love humanity demonstrated for Him. His focus was the love of his Father. In the survey alluded to earlier, the question was asked, "what is the Biblical concept of submissiveness?" The response to this question is illustrated in TABLE II.

SUBMISSIVE COMPARISON
TABLE II

Responses	% of sample
The wife is to be submissive to her husband.	55%
The husband is to be submissive to his wife.	0%
The man and woman are to be submissive to each other.	45%

Survey Question: What is the Biblical perspective of submissiveness?

Participants: 38

Types: Professed Christians, primarily leaders

Sex: Male 24%, Female 76%

Special Note: Submissive is exchanged for subject in some versions. The Greek word is the same for both words (Hupotasso).

As demonstrated by the illustration, the majority of respondents are persuaded that the Biblical concept of submissiveness is consigned to the wife. A closer look revealed that the majority of the men (66%) believed that the woman should be submissive, while the majority of the women (56%) believed in a mutual submissive relationship. And no one selected the husband as being submissive to the wife except in a mutual setting.

Based on the statistics reported, more than half the Christians in relationships or entering relationships either do not understand the concept, or will have a contrasting view to that of the spouse. This is an important point to remember.

The "Alternating Subject Command" is an imperative Christian concept applicable to all social relationships (Ephesians 5-6). Nevertheless, half the Christians are beginning marriage with differing concepts. This is the source for potential problems.

However, for those who understand the Alternating Subject Command, in addition to one's love for God, what else should motivate the husband and wife to accept such a command?

Wife's Command

The wife is commanded "to be subject to her husband as to the Lord (vs.22), because the husband is the head of the wife." Eph.5:22. Paul explains in I Corinthians Chapter 11 that headship is based on the fact that woman was made for man. He further explains that man is not independent of woman nor is woman independent of man (vs.11). Also, human rebellion began with the female (Genesis 3:6-7). Based on the "principle of origin," a rebellious spirit will be a principal issue facing women in the marital relationship. This is discussed in great detail in <u>Rebels and Tyrants to Husbands and Wives.</u>

The wife's reverence cannot be based on her husband's responses. She must be supportive of her husband because of her love for God. This is the only way that a relationship can continue through difficult circumstances. This does not mean that a person should remain in a life threatening or physically abusive situation. In such a case it would be wise to separate with eventual reconciliation in mind. The Christian's call is "forgiveness and restoration." The consequences of spousal abuse will be discussed in the chapter entitled, The Exception Clause, Limiting and Liberating.

Husband's Command

The man is to "love your wife as Christ loved the Church and gave himself for her (Eph. 5:25)." Jesus demonstrated unparalleled love and a sinless life. In response to a marital situation, which seems to be intolerable, the Scriptures guidance might appear to be unfair. In the light of the reply of unfairness one must always remember "Jesus." It was not fair that Jesus gave himself for us. His death for us in the midst of our sin can only be accepted by faith since it is beyond human comprehension. BUT HE DID IT. The command to the believing husband is that he is to love his wife likewise. Jesus' Greatness Principle is applicable here when he said, "the greatest in his kingdom is the one who is of greatest service (Matt. 9:35)." The husband is to be as a servant in his relationship.

The husband's love must not depend on how the wife responds. It is in spite of her responses to her husband's love. Again, the man's focus must be on God, not the responses of his wife.

Hindrance to Prayer Problem

Finally, in I Peter 3:1-7, Peter reinforces and confirms the writings of Paul. Please note verse 7, the husband and wife are joint heirs of grace. Each spouse should take great care of their relationship. There are special blessings just for the two. Peter warns the man to obey the command so that his prayers will not be hindered. Hindering often means to slow down, or to impede to a slower pace. The Greek word translated here is a combination of two words ek (from, out,) kopto (chop, or beat repeatedly), ekkopto. The emphasis of the word in the context of the verses is that the prayers are severely damaged as the result of the activities of the relationship. It is important to note that another Greek word closely related to kopto is temno. Neither temno or any of its derivatives are used here. In contrast to kopto, temno infers a single "decisive" blow. So, Peter does not mean that prayers are not heard.

When emotions flare due to marital difficulty, it is difficult to pray with a clear and unimpeded spirit. This is more likely the explanation of Peter's statement. When marital discord occurs it affects every aspect of the believer. Understandably, one's prayer life is affected.

In terms of the believers prayer life, spiritual growth, and daily living the status of such is dependent on the condition of the marital relationship. This is the meaning of Peter's "joint heirs." Whether the union is a believer to non-believer, or believer to believer relationship, the guidance is clear and convincing. The responsibility of the believer in a marital relationship is far greater than that of a non-believing counterpart.

A Study on Divorce and the Christian

Given the perspective on marriage, one might easily assume what the perspective on divorce would be. There are circumstances when, unfortunately, divorce may be a believer's alternative. Therefore, it is important to review a perspective on the Christian and divorce.

Jesus Discusses Adultery

Matthew 5:27 is a continuation of a discourse on obedience to the Law. Jesus begins with verse 17 speaking of murder. In verse 27, he begins addressing how a person can commit adultery.

Jesus' explanation of how a person can commit murder and adultery is obscure or very different from the normal events of murder and adultery (Matt. 5:17-32). Also the remainder of Chapter 5, verses 33-48 are on the same topic of fulfilling the Law.

When Jesus begins the conversation on adultery (verse 27), he is speaking of ways a person can commit adultery. Remember, he is not addressing divorce. He is addressing the acts that constitute adultery.

In verse 28, He reveals that lusting for a woman is one way. This was very obscure. Typically, the thinking was that the only way one could commit adultery was to actually have sexual intercourse with a married person. Jesus' point is that adultery is the act of making arrangements or pre-positioning oneself to bring a sexual fantasy into reality. See James 1:15. The word translated lust in Matt. 5:28 means to "assault" or "lay upon." Therefore, adultery is already committed when the "preliminary" activities begin.

The other way of committing adultery has to do with anyone divorcing his wife. If one divorces his wife and she remarries, he causes her to commit adultery, unless she was divorced for an immoral act (unfaithfulness in some texts). Therefore, if a man divorces her because of immorality, he is not causing her to commit adultery by divorcing her. But the issue here is not whether or not divorce is permissible if a spouse is unfaithful. The issue is, "how can a person commit adultery?" So in the context of these Scriptures, Jesus is not saying that a believer is advised to divorce for adultery. He is discussing ways of committing adultery.

Jesus Discusses Divorce

Matthew 19:3-12 discusses the issue or question, "Is it lawful for a man to put away his wife for every cause?" (See Duet 24:1-4).

Jesus' Answer (verses 4-6)

Jesus refers to the beginning of male and female (one male, one female) he continues, "For this cause a man shall cleave (Hebrew - stick too, hold to), (Greek - adhere, or stick like glue) to his wife." Jesus states in verse 5b, "the two become one flesh," he reemphasizes by restating in verse 6, "they are not two but one flesh."

Jesus answered their question about divorce in two ways. First, God created one man, and one woman (male, female). This was not only a holy creation, but also a holy numeric pattern (one man, and one woman). Secondly, he states a mystery. The two become one flesh. And he repeats, "they are no longer two but one flesh. How this takes place is as miraculous as Eve being created from the rib of Adam. When two people become married the flesh of the man becomes the flesh of the woman.

This type of mystery is not unusual for Christians. Another great mystery is when a person becomes a believer, the righteousness of Christ is extended or imputed to the believer (Rom. 4:19-24). Nevertheless, Jesus answered the question. The question is, how can one divorce his or her own flesh?

How can a man cut off his flesh and live without it? A person can live, but not as the person or couple they were during their marriage. It is a spiritual union that is encompassed in temporal flesh.

Jesus continues in verse 6b, "what therefore God has joined together let no man put asunder". Here is the catch. This is where the question is often asked, "what if God did not join the marriage together?" Jesus was talking to Jews, particularly Pharisees, and no Pharisee or religious leader would ever admit to marriage that was not sanctioned by God.

Nevertheless, one could still argue that the marriage was not ordained by God. And this would be a legitimate argument. It may be a marriage that God did not ordain. However, in the context of what Jesus is saying, he is not addressing what to do if the marriage was not ordained by God. He is addressing whether it is lawful to divorce. The Jews in his presence fully understood what he was teaching. IT IS TOTALLY UNLAWFUL TO DIVORCE. This is why they asked in the following verse, "Why did Moses then command to give a writing of divorcement?" They did not believe Jesus' answer. He had just told them two reasons why divorce was not lawful. First, in the beginning they were created male and female. Secondly, the two become one. They did not want to accept his answer. So they compared His reply to the Law of Moses (see Duet. 21:24, and 24:1-3). They asked, "why then did Moses command to give a certificate of divorce, and to put her away? (Matt. 19:9)"

Jesus answers, "because of the hardness of your hearts." A stronger word translated from the Greek is "because of obduracy."

This means, they were determined to dissolve their marriages. In verse 8b he makes reference again to what he has said earlier when he states," In the beginning it was not so."

They still could not understand what sin was committed by divorce. This is interesting. What is the sin one has committed if a person gets a divorce? There is no title for it. If a woman distorts the truth, she is lying. If a man takes something that does not belong to him, he is stealing. But what is it when a person divorces, if it is unlawful?

The apparent mystery of the sin was a problem for the Jews as well as the position, which Moses stipulated. They did not see any obvious sin. So in verse 9, Jesus shocks them with a sin that they all understood. He said, "Whosoever shall put away his wife, except it be for immorality, and shall marry another, committeth adultery: and whosoever marrieth her which is put away doth commit adultery." Clearly, Jesus demonstrates that these Jews could not negate the spiritual bond with their wives by giving a divorce decree. If they subsequently married another person such an act was adulterous; or if the divorced wife married another person the husband remains responsible for causing the adultery.

Adultery was punishable by death for both the man and woman (Deut. 22:22). Adultery was a sin against the nation. This is important to remember. They understood adultery. Since adultery was a criminal act and punishable by death, it would not be necessary to divorce a person because of adultery. Under the law it would be moot to divorce an adulterous husband or wife. The offender committed a crime against society like a murderer.

Therefore, the offender would be stoned to death. Much like the "woman caught in adultery (John 8:4)." In the case of the woman caught in adultery, Jesus grants her forgiveness. This is a point that is not to be overlooked.

The truth is that if Jesus forgives then we are to forgive. The principle, which Jesus exhibits by forgiving the woman demonstrates that adultery does not constitute an act necessitating divorce. A sincerely repentant spouse who asks for forgiveness and restoration does not present an option discretionary to the offended spouse. Forgiveness is a Christian imperative. Nevertheless, one of the overwhelming realities of adultery is that it is so damaging to the relationship, the offender should realistically expect a demanding rehabilitation process--even when the offended spouse finds the spiritual strength to forgive and restore. The length of such a process will depend on the spiritual depth and determination of both partners.

In terms of the legality of divorce, the act itself is not commended by Jesus. But since the Jews (Pharisees) could not understand the sinfulness of the act of divorce, Jesus addressed their subsequent objective of remarrying, which was adultery (i.e., where the exception does not apply).

The Exception Clause, Limiting and Liberating

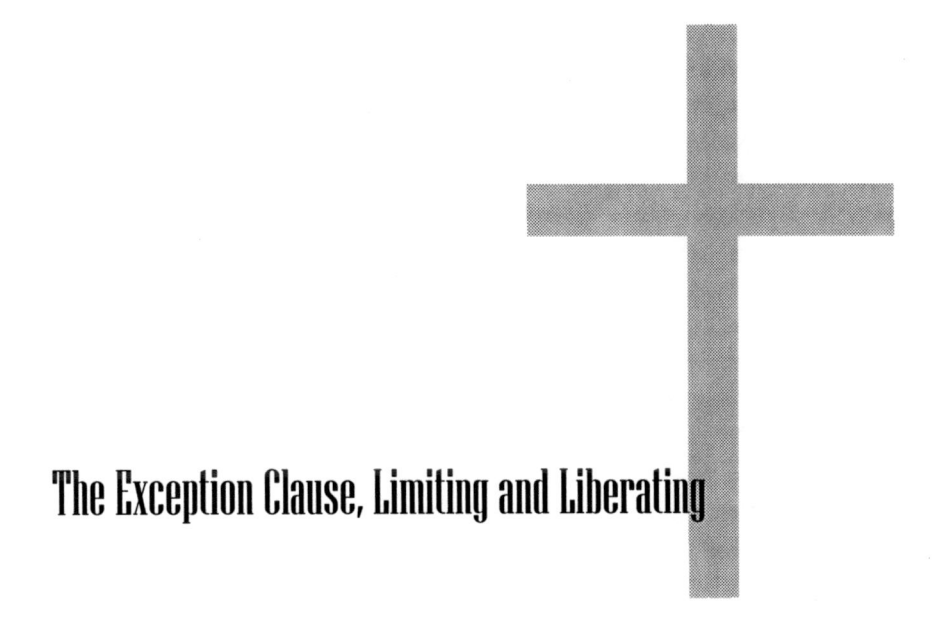

Limiting and Liberating

There is a wide spectrum of views on this clause attributed to the exception stated by Jesus. This guide evaluates this clause extensively. The author of this study poses some major challenges to typical views, and provides sound Biblical scholarship, logic and the influence of the Holy Spirit in expounding this section.

Understanding the Exception Clause

As shown in the previous chapter, the exception when divorce is warranted is when immorality is disclosed. There are several views on what Jesus means by immorality.

Typically, some scholars conclude that he means the spouse has committed adultery. And therefore, divorce is a viable and supported option. However, it is doubtful that Jesus meant that divorce was an alternative if a spouse committed adultery. First, The Greek word for adultery is different than the word translated immorality. No doubt, Jesus would have specifically said, adultery, if that is what caused the exception. Secondly, adultery was punishable by death. As a matter of Law, there would be no need to divorce an adulterous spouse. See Romans 7:22, I Cor. 7:39.

Some versions use the term, unchastity to circumvent the "adultery" problem as shown above. This is the violation when the husband discovers that his wife was not a virgin as told or assumed prior to marriage. Concerning the Law, if a man discovered such a breach of relationship he could bring his wife before the elders. However, this view has the same flaw as those who believe adultery is what Jesus intended as the exception. Again, a woman who was found guilty of such an offense would be stoned to death. As a matter of Law, divorce would be moot. In fact, if the husband alleged a wrongful accusation, he could never divorce his innocent wife. See Deu 22:15-21

Interestingly, most translators have discontinued the use of adultery or fornication as the translation for porneia. This is because of the rationale provided. The typical rendering of porneia carries sexual connotations. However, due to the evidence presented porneia or immorality represents an act or acts so deceitful and detrimental that the behavior clearly breaches the spiritual bond, and one-flesh covenant. In Matt. 19:9, the term porneia could not be adultery, lasciviousness, or other sexual sins which result in divorce by definition.

Straining to make the point that Jesus meant "adultery," Thomas Edgar (Divorce and Remarriage [Four Christian Views], pg 151) argues that porniea was used for a woman who commits adultery, and moicheuo is used for men who commit adultery. Moicheuo is most often translated, adultery. Edgar makes a glaring error by not providing an example of this grammatical idiom in the New Testament.

This view is further invalidated by the account of the women caught in the act of adultery. See John 8:3. She is accused of moicheuo not porneia. Whatever Jesus meant by porneia it is reasonable to conclude that it would not require death.

Therefore, Jesus' exception is an act or acts that would not require the death penalty, but the act or acts would be a cause to dissolve the relationship as a matter of Law.

Offences such as spousal idolatry or spiritual adultery where other persons, things or acts take precedence over the spousal relationship could be the type of violation in question. The metaphor or illustration of "harlotry" was often attributed to Israel for her idolatrous behavior and alliances with forbidden nations (Lev. 20:6, Num. 15:39, Deu 31:16, Jer. 3:8, Eze. 6:9, Eze. 16:28).

A classic example of spousal idolatry is a person who abandons the marital relationship. Paul discloses that believers should stay with non-believers if the non-believing spouse desires to remain married. Contrariwise, the believing spouse is not bound if the unbelieving spouse departs (I Cor. 7: 15). Notice, Paul states that believers are to stay unmarried or reconcile if they separate (I Cor. 7:10-11). However, upon separation, it is understood that either party must maintain their care responsibility to the degree possible. Unless, they separated due to a serious and repeated violation.

Fortunately, Paul provides additional insights to determine when a "confessed" believer is in fact an "unbeliever" or to be treated as an unbeliever. Paul discloses a serious indictment of persons whom do not provide oversight and the necessities for their families. Paul states, "they are worse than unbelievers." See I Timothy 5:8. This is a violation of "Principal Care." Clearly, this instruction to Timothy is to treat or classify such persons as unbelievers. Persons departing their relationships with utter disregard for the welfare of their families, fit the condition of an unbeliever in I Corinthians 7:15.

Conclusively, a confessed believer who departs or neglects his principal care responsibilities is considered an unbeliever. I prefer to use the descriptive term, "manifest unbeliever" for such persons. This person confesses to be a Christian. However, by virtue of neglecting one's family similar to abandonment, this person is "in-fact" an unbeliever. The innocent spouse would not be bound. Other possibilities include unrepentant physical battery, mental cruelty, and other wanton acts of disregard for family care (See the Biblical description of mental cruelty in the case of Mr. and Mrs. Harris, Chapter VII, A Matter of Repentance

Additionally, the person who does not hold family in high regard will certainly violate Matthew 19:9 spiritually if not physically.

There are those persons who would reject the view that Jesus Christ was also including spousal idolatry and spiritual adultery as outlandish and stretching to make a point. However, those persons are limiting the exception clause to mere physical acts. Jesus clearly illustrates that sexual immorality, and specifically adultery is not limited to the consummation of a physical act. See Matt. 5:28. It is a pharisaical presupposition that sexual sin is purely a physical act. Theologians and practitioners who limit the exception clause to sexual acts miss the efficacy of Biblical truth concerning relationships. God's purpose concerning believers is to create clean hearts. See Ps. 24:4, 51:10, Heb. 10:22.

Finally, why is it so difficult to reason that Jesus Christ would speak consistently with Old Testament form. After all, God was the first to describe Israel's behavior as adulterous.

Larry Richards in Divorce and Remarriage (Four Christian Views) admits, "the exception clause approach fails to address the nature of the unfaithfulness cited by Christ. The New International Version translation is unfortunate, but illustrates the confusion of scholars over the exact meaning of porneia." Richards continues later in his essay, "...attempts to define porneia do not seem to help us clarify Jesus' meaning. Is he speaking of some previous sexual sin of the divorced partner? Or is this simply an illustration of hard-heartedness in a marital partner? Or does Jesus imply a special class of divorce and remarriage cases? Our appeal to first-century Greek usage and Jewish custom leaves us with no certain answer."

It is clear in Richards' study "porneia" could have a wide range of meaning. While Richards' conclusions are different, his statement concerning porneia underscores my Biblical position concerning porneia's meaning. It could be sexual, attitudinal, spiritual or have other implications.

Thus, it is accurate to use the context of Jesus statement to describe an "immoral breach of relationship." This breach is witnessed in a number of Biblical illustrations. Again, Jesus is not stating that divorce is required. He provides the exception as the only Biblical rationale for divorce. The men and women offered as an example, violated the spiritual bond and care covenants of their relationships. Notwithstanding the reason or whether their spouses agreed, their motives were often self serving, and they clearly deceived their spouses or abdicated their "principal care."

Biblical Examples of Immoral Breach

Abram in Egypt

Given the command of God to depart his homeland on two separate occasions, Abram asked Sarai to explain to foreigners that she was his sister. While the typical believer glosses over this barely taking notice, the decision exposed his wife to great danger, and only God's intervention stopped what could have terminated "their" relationship. Perhaps the first occurrence was more understandable, but to witness God's intervention the first time and continue to expose Sarai was an "immoral breach of relationship." While not deceitful, it was clearly self serving and it could have resulted in grave consequences. Notice in both cases the men asked Abram, why did you do it? It is questionable whether Abram's life was endangered. He certainly thought that he would be in danger. Nevertheless, based on the facts of what occurred, Abram's life was not required. See Gen. 12:11-18; 20:2-16.

Isaac and Rebekah's Example
Isaac followed his father's example and led the people of Gerar to believe that Rebekah was his sister. The king witnessed Isaac and Rebekah playing with each other in a manner of a husband and wife. The king questioned Isaac's motive. As with Abraham, God's intervention rescued the relationship (Gen. 26:6-11).

Later in their relationship, Rebekah's scheme and deception subverted her whole family. She plotted and commanded Jacob to deceive his father, and extort Esau's blessing. It caused a cardiac episode in Isaac, and Esau was filled with murderous rage. Finally, Jacob had to depart in fear for his life (Gen. 27:5-33, 41-45).

Fortunately, in the cases involving Abraham, Isaac and their spouses the Lord used their weaknesses to accomplish His absolute will. It cannot be proven that God condoned their lies and deceit to accomplish His will. Both of these marital relationships continued.

Unfortunately, the following examples do not end with relationships intact:

Samson and His Wives
Often viewed as an undisciplined illustration of carnality, Samson proposes a wager with several men concerning a riddle, and an animal he destroyed. These men threatened to kill his wife's father if she did not explain Samson's riddle. She cried to Samson repeatedly without disclosing her true motive. Samson gave her his rationale for not telling her. He explained that he withheld sharing the riddle with his own parents. This is particularly noteworthy because it is the classic comparison of spouse versus parents. Eventually, Samson tells his

wife the riddle. Albeit, it was not because she was his wife, but he did elevate her above the status of his parents. However, Samson was demoralized when he discovered that she immorally breached their relationship.

Understandably, her father's house was threatened, but she chose to completely deceive her husband, elevating both her father's needs and the demands of other men above her husband's concern. Subsequently, Samson terminates the relationship. His wife's error may not appear to be a grave violation to the casual observer, but the deceitful, unfaithful, and insidious nature of her act destroyed Samson's bond and trust. Later, Samson attempts to reconcile with his wife, but she was given to another man (Judges 14:10-20; 15:1-2).

Delilah, while not identified as a wife provides an excellent example of an immoral breach. Similar to Samson's wife, she conspires with the Philistines to abate Samson's strength. She is successful, and Samson is rendered helpless against the Philistines. She was paid for her services. Regardless of Samson's lack of wisdom, Delilah demonstrates all of the characteristics of an immoral breach. She displayed harmful intent, deceit, and complete disregard for "principal care" (Judges 16:4-21). Whether or not Delilah was his wife is not the point. The conclusion is that one would expect such behavior from an enemy, not a wife, concubine, betrothed or fiancé.

The Levite and His Wife

Perhaps the most gruesome example of immoral breach happens in Judges 19:1-29, when a Levite along with his wife or concubine travel through Gebiah to Ephraim. While in Gebiah, they lodged at an old man's home for the evening. Some Benjamites in Gebiah beat on his door, and they demand that the man visiting be given to them for homosexual pleasure. The old man offered his own daughter and the man's wife. The men would not listen.

Meanwhile, the husband pushed--by inference--his wife out to them, and these men abused her all night. She died at the door step in the morning. Her husband severed her body into twelve pieces and sent her body parts to the other tribes of Israel. The rape was viewed as a corporate crime against Israel and a war ensued. But when asked to give an account of events, the husband did not explain that his wife was sacrificed to save his life. See Judges 20:3-5. Clearly, the act of placing her in "harms-way" would constitute an immoral breach on his part.

These are examples of a Christ-based Counseling view of what Jesus meant by the exception clause. The Jews and society at large had a long history of treating women like chattel. Only in situations where the spiritual bond, and one-flesh covenant is breached does Jesus cite as warranting divorce.

Excluding Isaac and Rebekah's experience with Esau and Jacob, each example has sexual implications or relations with other men or women. Each example involves deceit and unfaithfulness with grave circumstances. All involve a violation of "principal care" where the spouse was not given priority care and oversight.

These are examples of persons who illustrate an immoral breach. There are also examples of persons who could have breached their relationships. The following are examples of two women who honored their relationships under great duress.

Sarai's Example
Sarai followed her husband without knowing where she was going, and then she was called upon to protect her husband by saying he was her brother. She placed herself in jeopardy of loosing her husband, and becoming another man's wife. She did this on two separate occasions. No wonder Peter refers to her in his illustration of a godly woman. See I Pe. 3:1-6.

Abigail's Example
Abigail's husband placed her in a position where she and her whole household could die. Her husband, Nabal, insulted David and his men. David was determined to destroy Nabal's household. Abigal interceded and pleaded with David, and David changed his mind. Later, Abigal told her husband all that transpired concerning David's plot, and her husband went into shock from his own foolishness. Later the Lord terminated his life. Abigail did not breach her relationship, which she could have done. Although her husband was known as a foolish man, she honored their spiritual and one-flesh covenant. And she clearly demonstrated the standard of "principal care." See I Sam 25:1-36.

Exception to the Exception
The term, Exception Clause is the title given historically to Jesus' statement concerning acceptable conditions for divorce and remarriage. However, Jesus never used the term, exception clause.

All of the confusion surrounding the exception clause demonstrates how easy it is to become overwhelmed by the intricacies of the Law.

Contextually speaking, Jesus responded to a question from the Pharisees concerning the Law in Matthew 19:3-12. The question addressed the lawfulness of divorce. Interestingly, the Pharisees focussed on the lawfulness of divorce, but they were not concerned about the love required to heal and restore a relationship.

When considering the Law, there is an overriding principle that must be understood about the counsel of God. The Law is a contingency. God has provided contingencies on a "continuum" for man's circumstance. These contingencies flow from God's principal characteristic, love.

The Law does not always fit man's condition. Love exceeds and covers the human flaws, gaps, and ironies the Law is not designed to cover. This must be the overriding factor guiding any counsel concerning believers.

Biblical Illustrations of the Exception to the Exception

Does love take precedent over the Law? If so, is this clear in Scripture?

Adam's Sin

While the written Law did not exist, God's command represented an oral code with a penalty of death if violated. Adam violated God's command, and was consigned to death. God could terminate Adam immediately, but what we see in Adam's post-sin existence is a contingency. Additionally, the consequences of Adam's sin including his nakedness was covered. See Gen. 2:17-3:23. Where God's command could terminate Adam immediately, love provided Adam with life, covering, and reconciliation.

David's Sin

David's offense is one of the most chronicled atrocities in Biblical history. He commits adultery, and he concocts a murder plot that destroys the woman's husband and his support personnel in military combat. See 2 Sam. 11:20-24. David's "hidden" sin was explained to him in a concealed anecdote by Nathan the prophet. The anecdote told by Nathan described a rich man who took the only sheep of a poor man.

While the offense was criminal, it would not warrant death. Upon hearing the anecdote, David was filled with righteous outrage. No doubt, using the Law as his guide David proclaims, "As the Lord lives, surely the man who has done this deserves to die." Nathan told David, "you are the man."

Actually, David's judgment against the rich man in the anecdote exceeded the punishment rendered by the Law. However, David's crime warranted death. Both adultery and murder required the death penalty. Nathan's **reply** to David's overwhelming guilt and confession provides the governing principle for all human conditions.

The Scripture proclaims, "And Nathan said to David, *'The Lord also has taken away your sin*; you shall not die' " (2 Sam. 12:12).

The Law exposes and terminates, but love atones, heals, restores, and provides a new beginning. It is further noteworthy that while David endured heavy personal and familial penalties for his acts, he was not commanded to severe his relationship with Bathsheba.

Love is such an overriding factor, not only does Solomon come forth out of the bond between David and Bathsheba, but Jesus Christ is a descendant of this "adulterous" union.

Love is the Exception to the Exception.

When counseling God's people, love and love's family of principles must be the principal standard (e.g., reconciliation, restoration, patience, sincerity, etc.). Love covers a multitude of fault (1 Pe. 4:8).

Joseph, Mary's Husband

Joseph found himself in an extraordinary position. He was betrothed to a pregnant woman whom he had not known sexually.

The typical believer explains, "she was pregnant by the Holy Spirit." This response is correct, but by Law it does not matter. Lawfully, Joseph had Mary's life in his hands. One public proclamation and Mary would be stoned to death. Therefore, he desired to put her away privately. Obviously, Joseph concluded that a higher standard was in order. He loved Mary. Joseph was called to be Mary's betrothed because he was a devout man of love. So, he was determined to put her away, privately. Fortunately, there was an exception to his exception. An angel revealed to Joseph that the child in Mary was conceived by the Holy Spirit. If God says it is alright, it is alright. See Matt. 1:18-20.

David and the Holy Bread

As David fled from King Saul, he and his men were hungry. They asked a priest for food. The priest responded that as long as his men did not have recent sexual relations they could eat the holy bread. The priest recognized that David's need was primary, and the Law was secondary. Lawfully, the bread was reserved for priests. See I Sam. 21:3-5; Lev. 24:9.

Jesus makes this point to the Pharisees when He was asked about his disciples activities on the Sabbath. Notice, the question was about picking grain on the Sabbath. Jesus responds by showing that David ate holy bread reserved for the priests. This seems to be an apples and oranges comparison. Emphatically, the issue is not Sabbath days or holy bread. Jesus' objective was to demonstrate the relationship between the Law and the principle of Love. Jesus continues, "But if you had known what this means, 'I desire compassion, and not a sacrifice,' you would not have condemned the innocent." See Hos. 6:6; Matt. 12: 1-7. Jesus had made this same point previously. See Matt. 9:13. Compassion or love is a higher order principle than the Law.

David Remarries Michal

David's first wife was King Saul's daughter Michal. Eventually, Saul desired to terminate David's life without cause. David had to flee for his life. Subsequently, Saul gave Michal to Palti, and she became Palti's wife. After Saul's death David demanded his wife back, and they were reunited. See I Sam. 18:27; 25:44 and 2 Sam 3:13-14. The Law strictly prohibited remarrying a former wife. See Deut. 24:1-4. One might argue that David did not divorce her. So, this is why he is allowed to reunite with her. However, the emphasis of the Law is not the divorce. The emphasis is on the fact that she has been with another man (vs. 4). "She has been defiled." David can marry her because Love is above the Law.

David's Incestuous Wives

In contrast to his reconciliation with Michal, David elected not to have sexual relations with the wives his son Absalom defiled. However, David did maintain his "principal care" responsibilities for them. Clearly, his wives' incest was attributed to David's sin with Bathsheba and Uriah. See 2 Sam. 2:11. Furthermore, his wives were victims of Absalom's evil. See 2 Sam. 16:21-22.

Nevertheless, if David obeyed the strict requirements of the Law, his wives would be executed for incestuous conduct. See Lev. 20:11.

Legalistic and Clandestine Warnings

A focal point of the Christ-based Counselor is to provide balanced Biblical instruction. The Christ-based Counselor must avoid leaving the impression that God is depending on flawless performance before He provides care for the counselee. While there will always be an effort to understand God's Word, His response to our needs is not based on exegetical or behavioral excellence. Even when we do not make the right interpretation or decision, He loves us. We have the assurance that nothing can separate us from His love (Romans 8:35-39).

Conversely, the principle of compassion over sacrifice, or love over law does not mean that a spouse can use this truth for unrighteous gain. A person must not abandon a spouse or other family responsibilities to commit sin under the guise of love for something or someone else. Anyone doing so, will do so to personal peril.

Times of Struggle, Revisited

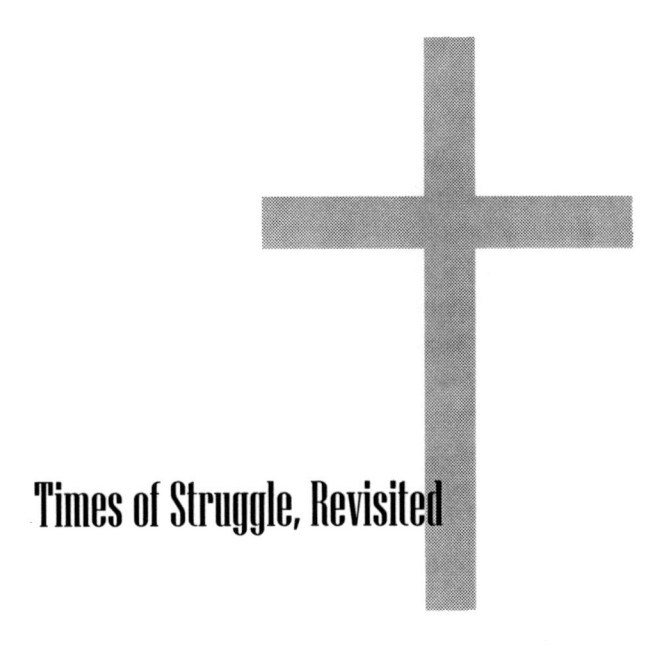

This section of the guide provides information on what should be considered from a spiritual standpoint for a Christian considering divorce. Although a perspective has been provided in previous sections, this section will evaluate those questions so often asked. This section also assesses the flood of accompanying thoughts and emotions experienced during the period of crisis.

Spiritual Problems

Given the previous Perspective of Christian Marriage as the basis for marriage, plain and simply divorce is a disobedient act unless immorality is cited as the cause. Such a statement can be difficult to accept in light of some horrendous situations which exist. It is reasonable to assume that every couple experiencing martial problems perceives their situation as the world's worst. However, there are believers bound in horrid situations.

Several case studies are provided throughout this guide as follows:

Ruth and Reginald Richards

Ruth has been married to Reginald for 20 years. They have two children. They are both in their early forties. Economically, they are middle class. They own a nice home and two automobiles. They have invested well over the years. Financially, they are solvent with no financial pressures. They started out at the age of twenty-one and have been together since that time. They were truly in love as a young couple, and financially they struggled during the early years of their relationship. However, they worked hard together and enjoyed their relationship during those years.

Both of them have Christian roots. They are both confessed believers. But as life became easier for them, they began to enjoy more of the world's pleasures and gave less attention to spiritual needs.

Years passed and it became obvious that the relationship was in trouble. Ruth was determined to guide the family in a more spiritual direction, while Reginald was fully enjoying life in its present condition. Ruth was becoming increasingly concerned about the spiritual welfare of the family, while Reginald became increasingly worldly. He began staying out late at night. He indulged in drugs and alcohol. He was obviously involved with other women. His disposition began to change until he was no longer the same person. His late nights became mornings, and sometimes he would not show for a day or two.

When he returned she would question him about his whereabouts. It was only a matter of time before Ruth threatened to leave. But each time he would appeal with great sorrow, and a repentant spirit. On occasion he would even return to church. This would last for a while, and then he would simply resort to his former behavior.

Ruth tried everything. It was common knowledge at her church because of her constant appeals to her pastor and close members at the church. She made attempts to enter counseling with him, which he never accepted. She entered counseling herself. She desired to uphold the Christian standard for marriage. For years she continued to encounter the same problem, and to date she remains in her current situation. Eventually, Reginald loss his job, and he experienced a lengthy period of unemployment. The mental and physical cruelty increased along with the financial instability.

This is an example of a horrible situation. We will use Ruth and

Reginald's example as our model for evaluative purposes. A question and answer section is provided to readily identify the particulars of this model.

Questions and Answers

1. Can the problems in the marriage be related to an act or acts of disobedient behavior? Yes, in practically every marital crisis, inappropriate spiritual behavior can be attributed to at least one of the spouses or both. Review Ruth and Reginald's situation and identify vices, habits, or attitudes which indicate spiritual problems.
2. What makes this such a difficult situation? Among other things Ruth lives daily with the following:
   - She deeply desires to maintain the Christian standard for marriage.
   - She is being physically and mentally abused, but she does not accept divorce as a Biblical alternative.
   - He has demonstrated that he has extramarital affairs with other women.
   - He uses drugs and alcohol.
   - She forgives him when he asks for forgiveness, and demonstrates a repentant spirit. She forgives him each time with the hope that he really will change "this time."
   - He always returns to his former behavior after convincing Ruth he has changed.
   - Ruth is living in torment. She lives daily in a situation which the average person would escape by means of divorce. But as painful as her experience is, she is equally convicted by her love and response to God's Word.
   - Reginald knows her position and conviction as a Christian. He uses this knowledge as a part of his plea when Ruth seems certain to separate.
   - Reginald lost his job. During a period when they should have experienced greater financial independence, they encountered a financial crisis.
   - Reginald will not leave.
   - In summary Ruth and Reginald are facing a host of

problems.
3. In light of Reginald's obvious infidelity, would seeking divorce be considered improper spiritual thinking? This is difficult to answer. Certainly, he has been unfaithful. But he asked for forgiveness. Ruth seems determined to forgive him. Remember, each time he asks for forgiveness, Ruth's hope is that "this could be it."

As illustrated in our model, the spiritual implications certainly make the issue of divorce one which exceeds the typical scenario encountered by an unbeliever. This is true even in a relationship as regrettable as the one offered as a model.

Nevertheless there are other issues as well, particularly the effect on the children, and fellow believers. The next section briefly discusses influence on others.

It is reasonable to suggest that in most cases when divorce is being considered, the possible effect on the children is weighed. However, the alarming divorce statistics involve millions of children[1] indicating that this is not considered as damaging as once feared. There is an often-used argument concerning the fate of the children.

Some people feel that it is better for children to live in a homogeneous condition with one parent, than to live in a dysfunctional environment with two parents. This is discussed in greater detail later.

The believer contemplating divorce must also consider who he or she is encouraging. That is, who else is going to use this divorce as the support needed to use the same method.

There are corporate issues involving others that the believer should be very concerned about when considering divorce. After all, the believer is "his brothers keeper." Nevertheless, for the purposes of this document two will be discussed, the children and the community of believers.

The Children

The case offered (i.e., Ruth and Reginald) is certainly the type of condition where any counselor would be tempted to recommend an immediate separation or divorce just for the children's sake.

When an individual considers any decision that will change the whole focus of his or her life, it is important to ensure that the extreme discomfort does not force the individual to think irrationally. For this reason, the aide of a counselor cannot be over emphasized. Sometimes, a friend or relative can be helpful if the friend or relative has not become so emotionally involved that he or she is unable to give sound Biblical advice.

This is particularly true in an evaluation of the effect of divorce on the children.

Sonja Goldstein L.L.B, and Albert J. Solnit M.D. have a different view of the concerns for the children of a frequently hostile marital situation. They report the following:

It is sometimes said that if a child has been surrounded by conflict his parents' divorce is in his interest because an environment of strife or incompatibility interferes with his sense of trust and gives him a distorted model of how people can get along in a long-term relationship. The child by this logic, is better off living in a tranquil single-parent home than in an emotionally divided two-parent household. But this is an oversimplification. One of the biggest threats to a child's security is the breakup of his family. While quarreling parents may distress him, this is in part because he anticipates and fears a family breakup, and it does not follow that the realization of his fear is easier for him than its continuance[2].

The reality of this statement is that there is great value in the structure of family alone. The structure provides a sense of safety, security, and significance for the children. Witnessing the removal, dismantling or replacement of one of the pillars is an experience far beyond the child's social realm. It affects the child's whole being (i.e., emotionally, socially, physically, etc.).

Nevertheless, the overwhelming statistics provide the assurance that children survive divorce. Often, this is the bottom line. They (i.e., the children) will make it. It is often said that children adjust better than adults. While this is an arguable statement, for the purposes of this document the statement is accepted. "Children adjust to new and varying situation better than adults."

Dr. Leonetine Young, in her book The Fractured Family states:

> The family has not lost its importance; it has lost its power and direction. It is needed more, not less, because now there is no other structure to fulfill that greatest of all needs, the development of a person. The school may teach

a child to read, but it cannot teach him to love. Book knowledge may produce scientific competence, but only life knowledge produces competence in living. Only the family can teach the most basic knowledge there is: how to live.[3]

The statement does not assert that a child cannot be developed in a single parent family. The facts demonstrate that children are developed under circumstances of this nature. The statement also does not infer that a child cannot learn love in such a setting. One would have to strain to perceive how children in the Richards' family could learn lessons of love. And Certainly, a child learns as much about the realities of living from the dissolution of a marriage as any other unfortunate experience in life. However, when considering divorce as an alternative, the individual must be aware of the actual concept being demonstrated.

A child can learn far more about the depth of true love in the Richards' experience, than can ever be demonstrated by the dissolution of the relationship. The greatest and most superior example of love on the human scale was demonstrated by Jesus. Jesus and those of us in the world for whom he gave his life are on absolute opposite ends of the cord of compatibility before accepting Him (I Pe.3:18). Resident in Him, we have the unparalleled example of light for darkness, good for evil, spirit for flesh, compassion for abomination, sinless-ness for sinfulness, reconciliation for rejection, love for hate. And through Him exists the possibility of demonstrating such a love (John 15:9-17).

Concerning knowledge about life, the concept taught a child in dealing with a problem through dissolution is simply to "dissolve it." Remove the thing that hurts. This is the quick and fast way of resolving the matter. When divorce is evaluated in terms of its mentality and commonality, divorce represents a form of insanity. Imagine using the same approach with a broken limb or any other wounded part of our anatomy.

Children need to learn the value of accommodation, understanding, forgiveness, long-suffering, patience, and the effect of prayer and obedience. And there is no greater forum to learn these virtues than during circumstances of interpersonal conflict.

The lesson that millions of children have been taught by divorce can be summed up in one word "escapism." Escapism occurs when a couple separate because one or both are looking for a different situation. This will be discussed later.

Whatever the decision, whether to remain in the relationship or divorce, it is universally agreeable that the children are innocent recipients of a calamitous situation. The decision rests with what is perceived as the lesser of two evils (i.e., the present family condition, or divorce).

The children are the most obvious of those affected by divorce. However, the actual effect is more ominous than one's immediate family -- particularly in the Christian Community and society as a whole.

The Christian Community

Our most readily apparent association with the Christian community is through the body of believers with whom we fellowship (i.e., the local church).

The dynamics of the fellowship of believers is an integral part of the Faith. We need each other. We are directed to demonstrate our love by caring, correcting, and sharing with each other. The fellowship is a full support system. When it is at its best, it serves every aspect of humanity (i.e., socially, physically, spiritually, mentally, etc.). It further stands to reason that we find individuals within the body who we admire.

It may be a pastor, deacon, teacher, director, musician, or simply a devout member. No matter how insignificant an individual may think of his or her contribution, there is mutual admiration among members. The Christian community is a family community inextricably united by the blood of Jesus Christ. When any part of the body hurts whether represented by a denomination, convention, local church, or individual, the universal body feels the results.

All this means is that every challenge we encounter individually is experienced by the Church. If a person falls, the Church does not fail, but it feels the effect of our personal failure. If a person sins, the Church does not sin, but the Church feels the effect of our personal sins. And if one divorces, the Church does not divorce, but it will certainly feel the effect of divorce. An examination of how divorce affects the Church is in order.

Individuals desiring to make a decision on any matter look for persons who have encountered similar situations. They evaluate the circumstances leading others to the decision, and they examine the results after the decision as well as other considerations. This is the natural process of an intelligent being. However, a degree of bias always exists. It is impossible to know the full and future consequences of any decision without the passage of time.

We are only trying to increase the probability of a positive outcome with our pre-decision analysis.

Nevertheless, the decision is based on what we can perceive. If we know that someone else has done it, we are more likely to do it. Unfortunately, what we see, or perceive may be a very small portion of the real situation. Herein lies the danger and reality of a decision to divorce. If a Christian decides to divorce, he or she will be used as a frame of reference for someone else to divorce. While no one can be fully blamed for the sin of another, we all bear the cross of influence.

Paul alluded to the principle of influence in several of his writings. However, his discourse on the incestuous brother gives full coverage to the issue of negative influence (I. Cor. 5:1-7). Paul is concerned that allowing such behavior will influence others who may consider similar activities. Furthermore, it is apparent that there was a sense of pride among some of the believers that they could tolerate such behavior. It was as if they had reached such a high level of spirituality, they considered the existence of the situation a demonstration of their superior spiritual knowledge. Paul instructs the Corinthians to excommunicate the brother. The action was with the hope that the brother would repent. The action would also minimize his influence upon others.

Obviously this was not a marital situation, but the principle certainly applies. More specifically there are two other situations, which serve to illustrate the effect a decision to divorce has on others.

There was a family of four brothers (the Thompsons) and all of them were married. They all were reared in a Christian home. However, only one of the brothers developed as a believer.

Ultimately, he became the source of pride in the family. He was the first to graduate from college. He became relatively successful with real estate investments, and in his professional career. He was a devout believer, and he directed his family in the same way he was reared. He separated after eleven years of marriage. He intended to dissolve his marriage. Interestingly, all three of his brothers were either separated or experiencing marital difficulties within months.

He personally feels at least partially responsible for the turmoil.

He was sought not only by his family members for morale support, but also by other believers considering divorce.

Another example of the principle of influence is on a larger scale. A pastor wedded eleven couples during a six year period. It was widely known that this pastor had major difficulties in his marriage, and evidence of extramarital affairs. Eventually, he divorced and remarried. The illustration below depicts the result upon the couples he wedded:

PASTORAL LEADER'S DIVORCE IMPRINT
TABLE III

Number	Status
2	Married, no evidence of major problems
4 (all 4 divorced after study)	Separated
5	Divorced

Nine of the eleven couples divorced. This would be an alarming statistic in a secular surrounding, it is unthinkable in a Christian environment. All of the couples know each other. And at one time, they belonged to the same fellowship. Why a situation like this is allowed to exist in a fellowship is a topic out of the purview of this document. Nevertheless, the influence on the fellowship would be difficult to deny.

While there must always be concern not to oversimplify any set of circumstances, the results of the two examples (i.e., children, Christian community) cannot be overlooked. While every man and woman is individually responsible for personal decisions, each believer must understand the dynamics of the fellowship, and more specifically the influence we have on each other.

The latter example does not present the same type of innocence as related to children of divorcing parents. But couples look for and should expect an earthly spiritual representative who holds high the virtues of the marital relationship. They were vulnerable to a misrepresentation of spiritual direction through the ministers acts. This had to have some degree of influence on their decisions.

In his book "David, After God's Own Heart", Dr. H. Edwin Young concludes a chapter dealing with David's act of adultery and it's consequences on his family as follows:

Mark it down! People all around can tell about the consequences of sin. Divorce is rampant in our society, and divorce is sin, as we all know-especially those who have experienced it. God can forgive, forget, cleanse, and put it under his blood, as he has for so many victorious Christians. But those same divorced people will testify about the consequences of that sin in the scarred lives of their children and of themselves. Sin can be forgiven, cleansed, forgotten, put behind God, buried in the ocean, but the consequences are there! The Bible teaches it, and we know it in life! Dissipate your life and God will forgive, cleanse, and try to restore you, but when your life organs have been damaged and your health has been destroyed, those scars, that consequence of sin, remains. Always! [4]

For Better or For Worse

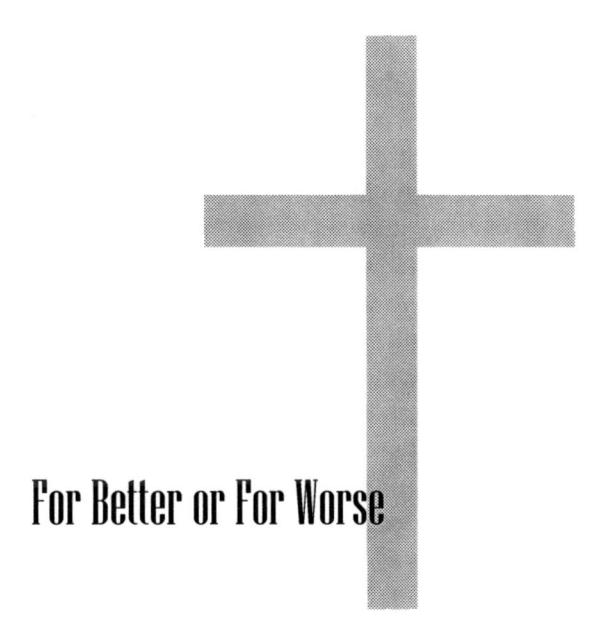

Divorce is a tragic event in the life of a believer. When divorce is being considered the counselee is weighing the appropriate decision under traumatic circumstances. This section of the guide is dedicated to the counselee's emotional and spiritual stability. This section of the guide addresses the emotions or attitudes the counselee may experience, and strategies to maintain emotional stability during this crisis period. Read very carefully, and make every effort to fully understand and apply the concepts provided.

The Principle of Renewal

Our emotions operate much in the same way as our physical system of feelings. The physical feelings we experience serve their greatest purpose when they warn us of impending danger. The damage that could be done if we could not feel the sensations of heat, or cold would be far more significant under such circumstances.

When we experience physical pain such as a stomach ache, it is a signal that something is wrong with the abdominal tract.

First, the signal informs us to evaluate what we have done to cause the problem, and secondly to provide the proper medication to alleviate it. If the pain continues over a long period of time, this could be a signal of a serious problem. The individual should seek the attention of a physician.

The emotional system operates similar to the physical system. However the sensors which signal problems are triggered differently. The individual with the stomach ailment actually feels pain in the abdomen. Several possibilities exist which could cause the pain, from consuming spoiled goods to stress. But the reality is that the person can feel the pain.

The person who responds emotionally to any of several experiences does so for different reasons from that associated with physical pain. Dr. Lawrence Crabb a noted Christian psychologist refers to the individual's basic assumptions comprised of all of the principles, experience, social mores, and other similar factors [1]. It is with this mental criteria that persons measure every event which occurs. However, there are other issues such as innate and spiritual influences that can cancel basic assumptions. This is the <u>Consummate Frame of Reference (CFOR)</u> *including basic assumptions, and innate and spiritual influences (Romans 7:17-24).*

An example of basic assumptions can be easily illustrated by marriage. Most people believe in the values of fidelity, monogamy, faithfulness, integrity, sincerity and other lofty expressions of one's commitment to another. And if a man or woman violates or is suspected of violating any of these values it will result in an emotional response by the spouse. The response will depend on the degree of importance attached to the principle violated. It could range from mild disappointment to homicidal jealousy.

An individual with a different set of values may not be affected at all by similar activity. During the course of time a prostitute either has never developed the same type of values, or has gone through a process of mentally deprogramming similar values (i.e., faithfulness, monogamy, sincerity, etc.). However, this does not mean that she cannot be affected emotionally. She simply has a different set of values or "mental packaging," which constitute her principles for living.

She may not believe in the virtues of monogamy, but she is a business person who believes in being paid for her services. She believes in the responsibility of meeting obligations, showing for appointments, and providing services "as agreed." And if she performs a service without being properly remunerated, an emotional response is guaranteed albeit for a different reason from the spouse who feels betrayed.

While this illustration is not to be construed as condoning prostitution, it is used to demonstrate the presence of an emotional and value system in each of us, and how this system varies from person to person.

The Consummate Frame of Reference can also be demonstrated. A wife denies her basic assumptions or signs indicating an unfaithful spouse. The fear of betrayal, or desperation to maintain a relationship cancels any clear indicators of an unfaithful spouse. Therefore, she readily accepts any explanation from her unfaithful spouse. This is one reason why people repeat mistakes. Their life-learned experiences are overcome by competing powers.

Crabb's premise is that a person can alter or change one's basic assumptions. However, the competing powers represent a much deeper and powerful challenge. Nevertheless, the response or answer is the same. God's Word can accomplish the task of changing one's perception about a given event, and empower the believer to respond victoriously. Therefore, memorizing Biblical truth is not enough. Clearly, it is a beginning, but the believer must sincerely pray for the Holy Spirit to make God's Word a living reality. The typical religious Sadducee or Pharisee was inundated with Biblical knowledge. However, most of them knew nothing of the power of God's Word (Mark 12:24, John 5:18, 39-40, 2 Tim. 3:5). Otherwise, the Biblical words have little value beyond intellectual or philosophical exercises.

Every time a counselor provides a believer with Scripture references in response to a crisis, emotional or otherwise, the believer is making an effort to invoke a different emotional response or view.

Crabb uses as his focal verse, "be not conformed to this world, but be ye transformed by the renewing of your mind (Rom. 12:2)."

However, in Chris-based Counseling, The Process of Being Made Whole is more robust and all-encompassing. The second principle in the Process, "Balanced Biblical Thinking" represents the renewing process. However, the other steps in the Process of Being Made Whole call on other factors that empower the believer beyond perception enhancement.

As a counselee functions in the Process that person will effectively alter one's whole perception of the event. Moreover, the person's circumstances could also be altered by the Process. Where Crabb's presupposition is one dimensional (i.e., changing perception of the world), the Lord can actually change one's circumstances, and not just a person's perception.

As the proper Scripture set is applied under the appropriate circumstances along with other spiritual techniques, the believer can overcome any experience. This is the essence of the Process of Being Made Whole.

The Christian is guaranteed relief. But this relief is dependent on each believer's adherence to the Process of Being Made Whole.

The point here is not to erode an individual of emotional responses such as grief, sadness, anger, etc. These responses are as important as the feeling of heat to the physical touch.

Obviously, a believer has a major problem when he or she reaches a point of insensitivity. Nevertheless, any prolonged state of an emotional response signals a deeper emotional problem.

The objective of this section is to assist the reader in maintaining a sense of emotional stability in the midst of a crisis. The possibility of a dissolved marital relationship and the activities, which lead to considering such a decision can certainly be described as a crisis situation.

Using the principles discussed above, a list has been provided to support the counselee in identifying the emotion or attitude being experienced. The exercises and Scriptures will follow the listing. While some of the emotions or attitudes are very similar, a condition or definition will be provided to distinguish differences. Biblical personalities who illustrate the emotion will also be provided. While each of the emotions illustrated are defined in terms of the marital relationship, they apply to other social relationships and conditions as well.

Emotion/Attitude	Condition/Description
Agony	The result of prolonged suffering. Usually characterized by insensitivity to the will of God on the part of a spouse. No degree of acceptance of God's will to the point of repentance evident, disobedient acts continue. The suffering spouse is in a position of sacrifice for the one who is acting out of the

	will of God. The suffering spouse may or may not realize that the disobedient spouse is helpless and that the disobedient spouse is critically ill (spiritually). Biblical Personality: Jesus at Gethsemane (Matt. 26:36).
Anger	Result of personal mistreatment, or violation of promises, vows, usually characterized by "belief" that deception has taken place. The violator is seen as someone who definitely knows better or should know better though this may not be true. Biblical Concept: Jesus and the money changers (Matt. 21:12).
Anxiety	Anxiousness, impatient with the current movement of events, accompanied by fear. Biblical Personality: Saul's odious performance of a priestly function. (I Sam. 13:8-14).
Bitterness	Where anger is evident usually in an emotional outburst or wrath, bitterness is defined as the long term or on-going result of anger. It is characterized by continued ill feelings as a result of the initial act which caused the anger, and is accompanied by tactics to "get even," "wrath or vengeance," even in mild forms. Biblical Personality: Saul's efforts to murder David (I Sam. 19).
Confusion	Inability to think clearly on a matter. Flurry of opposing, counter, unrelated and related issues being evaluated on a matter, accompanied by despair which is further perpetuated by the inability to think soundly or to determine the proper action to take. Biblical Personality: Disciples in the Upper Room discussing the reports of the resurrection of Jesus (Lk 24:36-38).
Despair	Usually the result of viewing a dire situation with no apparent end in sight,

	(hopelessness). Biblical Personality: The two disciples walking on the road after the death and burial of Jesus (Luke 24:13-21)
Embarrassment	The result of life's consequences, which expose negative aspects of one's personal life or associations to others. The feeling of embarrassment is particularly acute when such behavior would not be normally expected personally or by others. Unlike guilt where the individual made a decision to become involved in a regrettable act, embarrassment can be caused by persons other than the embarrassed party. Biblical Personality: David's sons Absolam, Amnon (II Sam.).
Fear	Expectation of bad, negative, or an undesirable outcome of forthcoming or current events/activities. Biblical Personality: The disciples during the storm on the sea, with Jesus on board (Mark 4:35- 40).
Frustration	The state of mind, which results from being on the verge of meeting or realizing a goal but the goal is never reached. Biblical Personality: David's desire to build a temple to the Lord (I Chron. 22:6-16).
Grieving	Usually a result of the conviction of disobedient acts. Coming to the realization of extent or depth of sin in one's life. Biblical Personality: Peter's Denial of Jesus, Judas' denial of Jesus. (Matt. 22:54-62; Matt. 27:3-5).
Guilt	Guilt is closely related to grieving, occurring as a result of being convicted of sin. But guilt combines the added humiliation and embarrassment that results from knowing that others have personal knowledge of one's regretful activities.

For Better or For Worse ■ 127

	Biblical Personality: Peter before Jesus after the resurrection (John 21:15-17).
Insensitivity	Callous attitude toward others, which is the result of sin on the emotional system. No lasting feeling of joy, peace, lack of compassion for the less fortunate. Can be the result of a sinful relationship such as adultery, or other on-going acts of sin. The emotional dependency on sinful relationships or acts have disoriented, distorted or perverted correct emotional sensitivity to one's own condition as well as to others. The greatest danger of this attitude is that it can be misunderstood as a superior spiritual threshold in the face of situations, which would usually call for an emotional response. A believer may feel that he is a spiritual soldier, unharmed emotionally by any event. Being a spiritual soldier means that believers continue in spite of the pain, and not that pain is eliminated. Jesus was compassionate, and even cried. But he continued his drive to do his Father's will. Biblical Personality: David's cry, return unto me the joy of my salvation, Saul, Judas Iscariot (2 Sam 12:1-9, Ps. 51:12).
Loneliness	Feelings of being by one's self in the matter. The only one relating to a particular problem or issue. No help apparent. One must do it alone. Biblical Personality: Jesus on the Cross (Matt. 27:45-46)
Procrastination (Spiritual)	A casual or cursory acknowledgement of incorrect behavior or disobedient acts. No realization of the imminent danger and destructive capacity of activities, which can only be reversed by immediate and severe action. Biblical Personality:

	Corinthians Incestuous Relationship (I Cor.5:6-13).
Sadness	Feeling of a great loss of possession, relative, friend, or relationship. Biblical Personality: Mary questioning Jesus about Lazarus (John 11:28-33).
Uselessness	Feeling that nothing is being accomplished, and one has no power to change the situation. Biblical Personality: Disciples' inability to remove demon from boy (Matt. 17:14-19).

An individual can experience one or a combination of these emotions during a crisis. Furthermore, an individual may be grieving as a result of some act of sin. Subsequently, the same person may begin experiencing anxiety attacks as the result of the lasting repercussions of sin or sins committed. As one might expect, overcoming emotional stress of this nature can be complex depending on any of several factors.

A complete process is required for an individual to maintain a level of survival and eventual recovery. Christ-based Counseling provides the framework for responding to most of life's crisis. Here, "Balanced Biblical Thinking" is expanded as the Renewal Steps during marital crisis.

The Renewal Steps

Where the Principle of Renewal was discussed previously. This section sets forth the Renewal Steps. The case of Ruth Richards will be used to demonstrate practical applications of each phase of the Renewal Steps as follows:

> **R**emember The Essentials Of The Emotional System
>
> **E**stablish the Goal
>
> **N**eutralize the Emotion or Attitude
>
> **E**nact the Strategy
>
> **W**ithstand, Under Attack
>
> **A**ctualize the Renewal
>
> **L**oop the Process

Fig. 2.

Each phase is discussed as follows:

Remember the Essentials of the Emotional System

The importance of the emotional system was discussed earlier in the Principle of Renewal. When an individual encounters an experience or crisis which causes an emotional response, the experience may be extremely painful. That is, it is a typical response. Using Ruth Richards as an example, it would be understandable if Ruth vacillated among a combination of emotions including anger, agony, bitterness, uselessness, and embarrassment.

Ruth must REMEMBER that experiencing those emotions are not problems in themselves. She is suppose to experience those feelings. Her emotions are performing just as designed. And much like a physical sense of pain, her emotions are informing her that something is wrong, and action must be taken to correct the cause of the emotional stress. Another important key to remember is that after the initial act or event, which initiates the emotional response, the individual (Ruth) will experience emotional trauma on an intermittent basis. Depending on subsequent events and other activities, the emotions will reoccur.

Establish Goals

Ruth must establish survival goals. Goals for Ruth during this period could be any of the following or a combination.

> Maintain an open forum with her husband.
>
> Manage all family business affairs during the crisis if possible.
>
> Ensure that the children continue their daily routines as unaffected as possible.
>
> Minimize disruptions to her employment.

Fig. 3.

Ruth must realize that this crisis is going to take every ounce of spiritual, physical, and mental energy in her being to reach her goals. It will further require a great deal of courage and major decisions on her part.

Neutralize the Emotions or Attitudes

Emotional responses are natural, but if the emotion is prolonged or extremely acute, then the result becomes problematical (Luke 9:57-62). The objective here is not to totally remove the emotion, but to control it. The first step is to identify the emotion. Secondly, Ruth is to drill constantly on the applicable Scriptures. As Ruth drills and remembers applicable verses in the Word of God, she will also need to ask God to empower and guide her through the experience. Daily prayer, and prayer on-the-spot as needed is imperative.

Enact a Strategy

Anyone desiring to weather the storm of a crisis must have a strategy. The strategy for some is simply to alter the mind with drug and alcohol, or some other emotional depressant. Others seek a new relationship to soothe the pain. Ruth must outline what she will do when she encounters emotional strain:

Identify emotion.
Pray daily and throughout day for strength.
Drill applicable Scriptures.
Contact counselor or support persons where available.
Refrain from any decision during emotional surges.
Request a time period of prayer from other believers (e.g., 40 days).
Increase attendance of Bible study, worship, similar activities.

Fig. 4.

The strategy here is two fold. First, every effort is made to saturate oneself with every spiritual instrument available. Secondly, it is Satan's desire to destroy the mental health of any believer. And his operation will refrain from being the force behind prolonged mental anguish when he discovers that the individual is becoming more spiritually dedicated (Matt. 4:10-11; Luke 4:10-13). Resist the devil and he will flee from you (James 4:7b). Resist means to do the opposite of what Satan expects. When a believer responds to difficult circumstances with persistent prayer, praise, and determination, Satan's objective to shatter the believer's peace and mental-health is defeated. This does not mean that he will completely stop. He will have to flee and return later (Luke 4:13).

Withstand, Under Attack

Based upon the applicable Scripture (Eph 6:13), Ruth must have the full confidence that she will overcome the situation. She will be particularly susceptible to emotional strain during periods when she is alone, or when she is not thinking of anything else. It is during these periods that Ruth must concentrate on applicable Scripture. She must not "dwell" on events, which have caused her emotional discomfort (Phil 4:4-9).

Obviously, there will be times when she needs to reflect on the disclosure of events in order to make decisions to improve the situation. But she must not dwell on events, which can only deepen wounds.

When she feels the emotional stress, she must concentrate on applicable Scripture -- even to the point of repeating them out loud if necessary.

She will require the mental constitution of a warrior. She may be wounded, but she must continue to press forward in the battle.

Actualize Renewal

The mere fact that Ruth has a plan in place means that she is being renewed. As she succeeds through each period of emotional stress, she must recognize that she is being renewed. The very fact that she is preparing and prepared for the battle means she is being renewed. Ruth must see the renewal taking place. She must actually see herself getting closer to God as a result of this crisis. She is gathering positive results from a very negative situation. She is living in the reality of Romans 8:28-29. Every crucial human experience is a Christ-conforming experience.

Loop

Looping is an old computer processing term. It refers to a function in a computer program, which does the same thing continuously until a particular task is complete. This is precisely what Ruth must do. As she experiences renewal, she must maintain her strategy with all diligence. Often, an individual will experience relief through such a strategy only to enter another crisis because he or she did not stay in the loop. Conversely, computer programmers become very concerned about endless loops, because an endless loop will not allow the computer program to perform other functions. But for the believer an endless loop in the renewal experience would be a welcomed crisis indeed.

Summarizing, the person who is to survive the pain of the situation needs every positive advantage available. While other alternatives may be available, the individual must be sure that the strategy is wholesome.

The term, for better or for worse has become merely a philosophic expression in most cases. It seems that few people have the depth of concern, which Ruth Richards demonstrates. She is to be commended for her zeal. However, like other people who so often wrestle with their spiritual obligation in similar circumstances, Ruth needs clear spiritual guidance. It could be that even more drastic measures will be necessary for Ruth.

A Matter of Repentance

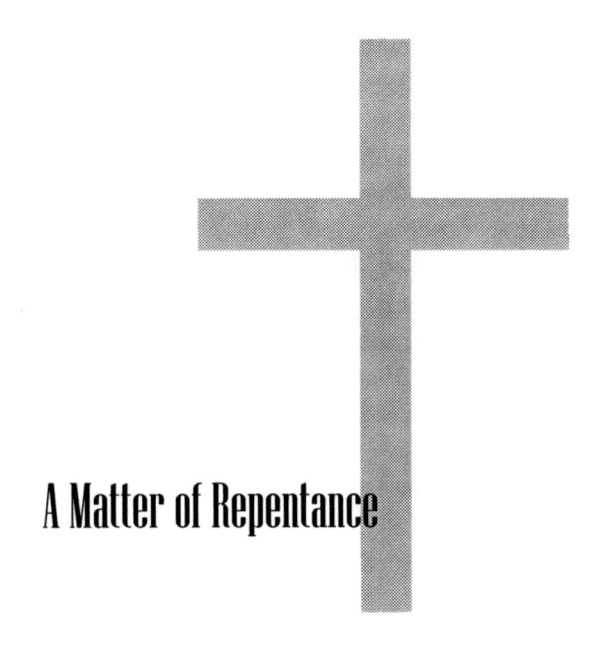

As demonstrated in previous sections, there are only two events, which can constitute divorce (i.e., abandonment by an unbeliever or manifest unbeliever, and immorality). Ruth's dilemma is primarily that she has a husband who has claimed to be a Christian. He also asks for forgiveness and shows brief signs of improvement. She knows that she must forgive him, when he asks for forgiveness. But he continues to repeat his offenses. Even with the best strategy and spiritual dedication, the torment of living under such conditions on a daily basis is taking its toll on her. Is Ruth spiritually obligated to remain in such a dire situation?

Physical Abuse, Mental Cruelty, Drug Abuse and Adultery

Again, there are many factors to be considered. But given the information as provided in the model (Ruth and Reginald Richards) two things are quite clear. Physical abuse not only offends spiritual laws, but is against the civil and criminal laws of the land. And this type of activity warrants no less than a separation if it is done with any regularity or irregularity.

Mental cruelty is as damaging as physical abuse. Craig and Clara Harris were married for almost 10 years. Clara had an emotional illness requiring hospitalization. She recovered in the subsequent years, but Mr. Harris desired a divorce. Mr. Harris committed acts against Mrs. Harris which bordered on criminal conduct. Mr. Harris staged domestic mishaps with the objective of causing the reoccurrence of Mrs. Craig's previous emotional problems. He would hide items from her (e.g. purse, important papers, etc.), gave her erroneous information and other such tricks to give her the impression that she had "lost her mind." One day he went so far as to point a loaded gun at her head, and threaten to kill her. Again, this type of cruelty is against civil and spiritual laws and should not be tolerated in any marriage [1]. A separation, or granting of divorce would be supported Biblically on the grounds that he requested it. And though he confesses to be a Christian, the wanton disregard for the life of his own flesh (i.e., his wife) makes his confession spurious at best. And while it is not impossible that a believer may become involved in such acts, the believer will not remain in such a condition. A spouse who displays such behavior can expect to face the lasting results of his or her actions [2]. Since mental abuse has become a common and misused allegation, the Harris's example serves as a standard of mental cruelty. One Biblical description of cruelty is merciless acts usually reserved for enemies (Exo. 6:9; Pro. 11:17; Jer. 50:42, Lam. 4:3).

Drug and Alcohol abuse are not as extreme as physical or mental cruelty. However, very often the physical and mental abuses are related to chemical dependencies. Nevertheless, illegal drug usage is against both civil and spiritual laws. And while a spouse may be more tolerant in this area, among other problems the tolerant spouse becomes the accessory to a crime to allow illicit drug use in the home (e.g. marijuana, cocaine, etc.). A separation should be considered in such a case.

Alcoholism has been defined as a disease, and consistent with any disease the ill person must be willing to seek the proper professional attention. The alcoholic is often irresponsible, unreliable, and disrespectful. And even when the alcoholic controls these aspects of his life, the physical damage to the body is undeniable. This should be a major concern to the spouse for the sake of the alcoholic spouse and the family.

Since corporal punishment is not administered in adulterous cases, adultery is a cause for divorce. And this was directly stated by Jesus. As shown Biblically in John 8:4, Jesus forgave the woman caught in adultery. And as stated earlier, certainly we must possess the ability to forgive likewise. However, adultery so violates the principle of one flesh, it rises to a level of contemptuous arrogance before God. Our adultery is a reminder of the adultery He suffered with Israel (Hosea).

When making reference to the women caught in adultery, it must be remembered that Jesus' final words were "go and sin no more." Earlier in ministry I had difficulty understanding that statement. I knew that there was no way the woman would not sin again. And certainly Jesus knew this, so what did he mean?

I'm Sorry, Forgive Me

The woman caught in adultery faced death as the result of her adulterous activity. It is difficult to imagine being in an electric chair, or gas chamber with the executioner's hand positioned on the switch. What was her thinking at the time when she was taken captive? Certainly, she heard or witnessed someone stoned to death because of similar violations of the Law. And now, here she was the victim of her own immorality. She was doomed to face death by stoning. But what a turnabout, the Master was there. The One who can forgive sins, and through His efforts she was given new life.

If she truly accepted and appreciated Him as her Savior -- and the value of her own life -- she would never commit such a grave mistake again. Jesus not only saved her from the eternal implications of her sin, but also from the earthly consequences of her sin. If she sincerely repented for subsequent acts of adultery, Jesus would forgive her, but she probably could expect to experience the earthly consequences of her sin (death).

Regardless of the excuse (e.g. vice, habit, dependency, addiction), or Reginald's explanations, Ruth is not to tolerate at any level of on-going acts of adultery including: flirting, staying out late, unaccountable whereabouts, and similar activities. The Spirit will not allow any believer to practice such behavior without grave consequences (I. John 3:9, I. John 5:16b). And if an individual continues, such a one has not repented, but has only said "sorry" as a shallow courtesy.

Often, when an adulterous spouse says sorry, what he or she really means is "whoops, sorry you caught me." The offender may beg, and even change briefly. But because of the insidious, and habitual dependency on the extramarital relationship, the offender longs for the other person's company. The adulterous activities continue in some form. Godly sorrow leads to permanent change (II Cor 7:10).

The Daniels were a couple who had separated for a period of time. As so often happens, both Mr. and Mrs. Daniels became involved in extramarital affairs during their separation.

Regardless of their excuses, or explanations, this activity constituted the absolute degradation of their relationship. This further highlights the danger of separations (I Cor 7:5).

However, they both reached a point of repentance, and decided they would reconcile. They both confessed that their extramarital relationships were over. Mr. Daniels who had repented of his affair first, realized the full effort involved in sincerely clearing oneself (i.e., spiritually, physically, emotionally) of such an affair.

And he was willing to support Mrs. Daniel as she went through the emotional withdrawal pains of a severed extramarital relationship.

However, Mrs. Daniels continued to maintain contact with her adulterous companion, and was simply unable to maintain her renewed commitment to her husband. While she was sincere in expressing fear that she would not be able to uphold her new commitment, such sincerity falls short of the true repentance necessary – particularly for an individual living in such a depraved condition.

Others reach a point where they will not even say sorry anymore because they know there will be a next time--or may be a next time. Still others say, I will try to do better.

All of these answers may be virtuous in terms of sincerity, but they are all the wrong answers for a matter such as adultery.

Can anyone imagine the woman facing death replying to Jesus, "I will try to stay away from him Jesus, but you know I am weak, and he and I have had some marvelous experiences. How can I stop this relationship!"

JESUS said "go, and sin no more". If Jesus' limit was that she must not commit such an act any more, then we are to do likewise. And if she was fully sorry, it would be very evident that she meant business.

Richard L. Strauss states in his book, Win The Battle For Your Mind:

There is a great deal of information in Proverbs about the right and wrong use of sex - what is wise and what is foolish. For example, 'But whoso committeth adultery with a woman lacketh understanding; he that doeth it destroyeth his own soul' (Prov. 6:32 KJV).

The word translated 'understanding' is the Hebrew word for heart or mind. He is out of his mind. He does not have any sense. He is not using good judgment. He has chosen a surefire way to ruin his life.

While the verse is addressed to the man (probably because he is most often the aggressor, the one on the prowl, who is looking for opportunities to satisfy his sexual desires), the same thing is true for a woman.

It is just as stupid for her to commit adultery. And it is not uncommon for a lonely woman, hungry for companionship and affection, to set herself up for illicit sex.

People who have been there know that what God says is true. They thought they had to get involved in order to meet some need in their lives. But committing adultery has destroyed them just as God said it would... It has built suspicion and distrust. It has sabotaged satisfying sexual relationships within marriage. It has alienated people from each other and instigated conflicts. It has caused disease. It has given children a negative model to follow and an excuse to sin. It has ruined Christians' testimonies before the world.[3]

What About Reginald Richards

If Reginald Richards is truly repentant there must be consistent and obvious evidence. He is going to do everything possible to make sure that he is accountable for his whereabouts. He may be more willing to participate in counseling. He may become involved in church activities to a greater degree than ever before. There are many other ways as well. It is his responsibility to demonstrate the sincerity of his repentance by deed. The life of his family depends on it. Whether or not his family survives as a single living entity depends on the depth of his conviction to overcome his behavior.

It is Ruth's responsibility to forgive him, and to recognize his efforts. So often an individual is sincere in repenting. But the offended spouse rarely recognizes the offenders efforts, and continually reminds the offender of the violations committed in the past. This indicates a serious spiritual problem by the unforgiving spouse, and it will never permit the relationship to heal.

Ruth and Reginald can expect a difficult road ahead, but with both husband and wife totally devoted to overcoming their crisis, with Christ as the foundation of their relationship, they will overcome the impossible.

Determining Spiritual Obligations

While all of the cases presented in this guide are extreme, this was done to demonstrate the severity that should be present before an individual considers separation or divorce.

Also, there are many other factors, which affect the relationship used as an example in this section of the handbook. While Mrs. Harris' situation warranted separation, could she financially afford it? And what about her children? Mr. Harris was determined that he would have custody of them.

Nevertheless, the objective of this section is to make it clear that Ruth Richards had no need of feeling spiritually obligated to remain in such a diabolical situation. She may opt to stay for other reasons, but she could not make a claim that she was spiritually bound to such a situation.

In fact, she may be the obstacle preventing her husband from reaching a point of true repentance. Given the case of the incestuous relationship in I Corinthians 5, Paul's instruction was that this sex offender would be excommunicated. It was the final act with the hope that the offender would realize the depth of his depravity.

What Ruth must realize and anyone else in the same situation is that to violate her is wrong, but Reginald's actual problem is with God. If he cannot honor and obey God's instructions, or repent then he is to be left to Satan (I Cor. 5:5).

Since she remained in the situation, Ruth began to resort to violent acts to protect herself. She was vulnerable to the impulses of her emotions and a sense of self preservation from his potential violence. Her own Christian character was severely jeopardized. The yeast definitely affects the whole lump (I Cor 5:6).

When an individual repents, the person not only experiences a deep sense of grieving (see Identifying Emotions Or Attitudes), but the offender takes positive and undeniable steps. The offender turns away from such activity and proceeds on a righteous path (Heb. 12:11-13). And if this type of repentance is not evident, the individual has not said, "sorry, I will not offend you in such a manner again." The person as actually said, "sorry, I'll try not to let you catch me the next time."

Final Thoughts

Figure 1, The Model of Involvement demonstrates the practical keys for a couple desiring to maintain the buoyancy and vitality evident in the Days of Wine and Roses. What so often happens in relationships is that they are taken for granted. The romance is gone. There are no more new horizons or surprises in the relationship, other than those, which destroy the relationship.

Where possible and to the degree possible, the couple should maintain those traits, which caused them to fall in love in the first place.

This of course is a simplistic view of a very complicated matter involving changes in age, social awareness, economics, family responsibilities, and other elements.

Upon the earliest signs of problems, a couple should seek Christ-based Counseling and other spiritual support groups. It is highly recommended that couples seek premarital counseling. They should maintain a counseling schedule in the same way regular medical check ups are approached. There are regular family seminars, and marriage conferences that should be attended regularly.

The effect of divorce on our society is undeniable. And the effect of Christian divorce even more disparaging. Each believer should be taught God's perspective on the matter regardless of the marital status.

Too often marriages are performed in our churches with minimum emphasis on the depth and spiritual implication of the institution. The clergy bears a major responsibility to inform believers about the seriousness of the divorce issue on the Christian Community and society as a whole.

If we are to overcome this demonic instrument of destruction, we must teach, train, and provide the best spiritual direction possible. Herein lies one of the underlying reasons for this guide. If it can prevent at least one divorce, or if it serves to provide relief and clear guidance when divorce is inevitable, it has performed as designed.

Notes

Preface

1. Andrew J. Cherlin, Marriage, Divorce, Remarriage (Harvard, Connecticut: Harvard Press, 1981)
2. Ibid
3. Ibid
4. Ibid
5. Ibid

Chapter I

1. United States Census Bureau, Number, Timing, and Duration of Marriages and Divorces: 2001 (February 2005)
2. The Barna Group, The Barna Update, Born Again Christians Just As Likely to Divorce As Are Non-Christians (September 8, 2004)
3. Ibid

Chapter V

1. Andrew Cherlin, Marriage, Divorce, Remarriage (Harvard, Connecticut: Harvard, 1981)
2. Sonja Goldstein, Divorce, & Your Child (New Jersey: Yale University Press, 1984)
3. Leontine Young, The Fractured Family (New York, New York: McGraw Hill, 1973)
4. Edward H. Young, David After God's Own Heart (Nashville, Tennessee: Broadman, 1984)

Chapter VI

1. Lawrence J. Crabb, Effective Biblical Counseling (Grand Rapids, Michigan: Zondervan, 1982)

Chapter VII

1. Gary R. Collins, Christian Counseling (Waco, Texas: Word Books, 1980)
2. Richard Strauss, Win the Battle for Your Mind (Neptune, New Jersey: Loizeaux Brothers, 1986)

Bibliography

1. Adams, Jay E. Christian Living in the Home. Grand Rapids, Michigan: Baker Book House, 1972
2. Aldrich, Joe Secrets to Inner Beauty. Santa Ana, California: Vision House, 1977
3. Ambron, Sueann Robinson Child Development. San Francisco: Holt, Rinehart and Winston, 1978
4. Bontrager, G. Edwin Divorce and the Faithful Church. Scottsdale, Pennsylvania: Herald Press, 1978
5. Bustanoby, Andre But I Didn't Want a Divorce. Grand Rapids, Michigan: Zondervan, 1978
6. Babbie, Earl R. Survey Research Methods. Belmont, California: Wadsworth, 1973
7. Collins, Gary R. Christian Counseling. Waco Texas: Word Books, 1980
8. Crabb, Lawrence J. Effective Biblical Counseling. Grand Rapids, Michigan: Zondervan, 1982
9. Cherlin, Andrew J. Marriage, Divorce, Remarriage. Harvard, Connecticut: Harvard, 1981

10. Daniels, Elam J. How to Be Happily Married. Orlando, Florida: World Publishers, 1955
11. Dobson, Larry Hide or Seek. Old Tappan, New Jersey: Fleming H. Revell, 1974
12. Fisher, Fred 1&2 Corinthians. Waco, Texas: Word Books, 1975
13. Goldstein, Sonja Divorce & Your Child Yale, New Jersey: Yale University Press, 1984
14. Hunter, Brenda Beyond Divorce. Old Tappan, New Jersey: Fleming H. Revell, 1978
15. Kerlinger, Fred N. Behavioral Research. New York: Holt, Rinehart and Winston, 1979
16. Lahaye, Tim & Bev Spirit Controlled Family Living. Old Tappan, New Jersey: Power Books, 1978
17. Morris, Leon The First Epistle of Paul to the Corinthians. Grand Rapids, Michigan: Wm. B. Eerdmans, 1976
18. Mumford, Bob The Purpose of Temptation. Old Tappan, New Jersey: Fleming H. Revell, 1971
19. Orr, William F. I Corinnthians. Garden City, New York: Doubleday & Company, 1976
20. Peppler, Alice S. Divorced and Christian. St Louis, Missouri: Concordia, 1974
21. Plekke, Robert J. Divorce & the Christian. Wheaton Illinois: Tyndale House, 1980
22. Rickerson, Wayne E. Getting Your Family Together. Glendale, California: Regal Books, 1976
23. Small, Dwight Hervey Design for Christian Marriage. Old Tappan, New Jersey: Fleming H. Revell, 1969
24. Stevens, Edward The Morals Game. New York: Paulist, 1974
25. Strauss, Richard L. Win The Battle For Your Mind. Neptune, New Jersey, 1986
26. Waylon, Ward O. The Bible in Counseling. Chicago, Illinois: Moody, 1977
27. Warren, Richard Answers to Life's Difficult Questions. Wheaton, Illinois: Victor Books, 1986
28. Wasserstrom, Richard Today's Moral Problems. New York: Macmillan Publishing, 1975
29. Weiss, Carol H. Evaluation Research. Englewood, New Jersey: Prentice Hall, 1972
30. Wright Norman The Fulfilled Marriage. Irvine, California: Harvest House, 1976

31. Young, Edward H. David, After God's Own Heart. Nashville, Tennessee: Broadman, 1984
32. Young, Leontine Fractured Family. New York, McGraw Hill, 1973
33. Zimbargo, Philip G. Psychology and Life. Palo Alto, California: Scott, Foresman and Company, 1977

Liberation and Deliverance Therapy
A Christ-based Counseling Perspective

Preface

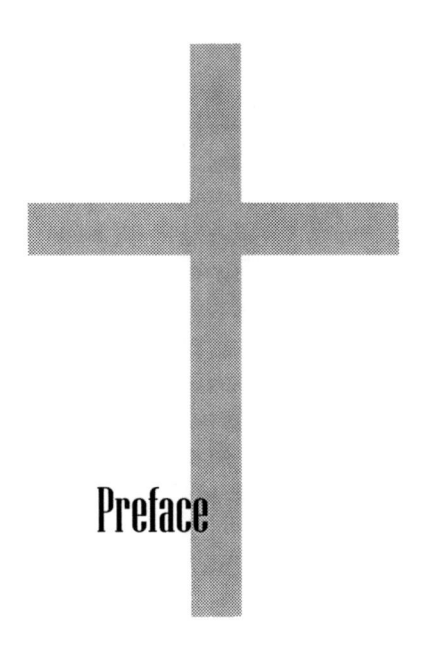

One of the most difficult conditions faced by a Christ-based Counselor is counseling persons who suffer with an addiction. Christian-based Counselors must possess an in-depth understanding of addiction from a Biblical perspective. A basic rule of thumb is that an addiction must be resolved before any other counseling concern can be addressed. That is, if the original counseling issue was marital, and the counselor discovers that one or both spouses suffer with an addiction, the addiction must be resolved first or addressed simultaneously. This is necessary because typically, addictions progressively dominate and control a person's life. This will be explained further in this counseling guide.

This guide is dedicated to believers who suffer with some form of addiction. Understandably, it is popular to offer specific programs and theories for specific addictions. Biblically, addictions have the same root cause, which will be discussed in detail. Obviously, there are differences in recommendations depending on the type of addiction being experienced. As an example, a person suffering with a substance related addiction might require medicinal support. However, a person suffering with an addiction unrelated to a substance does not require such support. Nevertheless, the root cause is the same regardless of the addiction.

Addiction is so pervasive that no one is immune. If we do not personally suffer with some form of addiction, most believers know persons who do. I am no different in this regard.

Yvette is a believer who admittedly has battled with substance abuse since she was eleven years old. She explains that she did not know what she was doing as a child. Her story is one of sexual abuse as a child, and a life of partying and progressive drug use. During this period she was raped, and exposed to a number of other abuses. When she became twenty-three, she received the Lord as her personal savior. She has continued to battle drug addiction. There have been times when she has been clean only to return to her addictive behavior. As of the writing of this document, Yvette has been clean for severa years.

I have a brother Chuck, who is an alcoholic. He has battled addiction for more than twenty years. He tells the stories of where alcoholism has taken him. He has entered in-patient programs on a number of occasions, and he is yet to break the shackles of alcoholism.

It is noteworthy that whenever examples of addiction are discussed, it is usually substance related addictions. Obviously, the difficulty to overcome such addictions and the accompanying damage warrants such coverage. However, this guide does not view substance-related addictions as the most widely suffered or most damaging addictions.

Later in this guide, a description of addiction is provided. Based on the description, the most damaging, far reaching, and insidious addiction is sex related. The societal devastation related to our inability to overcome or control sexual addiction relates to every other social problem.

Sex addiction affects humanity in general. However, it is currently a national crisis of "Biblical" proportions. One cannot avoid the daily barrage of sexual innuendoes, reminders, overtones, and undertones. This is evident on television, radio, news papers, magazines, and the internet. A hideous and ominous slogan explains the condition, "sex sells."

Where the typical believer cannot relate to substance related addictions, the typical believer can relate to sex related indiscretions. Notice, how I referred to them as "indiscretions." This is a pleasant and deceptive label for the most devastating addiction known to humanity.

When the issue of sex is discussed as an addiction, the overwhelming majority of us enter the picture. Regardless of age, gender, or marital status, most believers are vulnerable.

This guide uses sexual addiction as the basis for in-depth evaluation of addiction, and programming to overcome addiction. The Christ-based model provides for applications of Biblical truth to contemporary circumstances.

After studying this guide, there can be no doubt that terms such as "mental arguing" and "addiction threshold" capture the addict's personal struggles completely.

Fortunately, God's Word has the answer to addiction, and this guide is dedicated to the Yvettes, Chucks, countless believers, and your's truly who need this Christ-based Counseling approach.

Counselees must understand that while the Biblical illustrations in this guide are found in the Old Testament, the Old Testament illustrations provide the characterization of Jesus. While Moses is known as the deliverer, Jesus is the liberator, "consummate." Jesus is the deliverer, "consummate." As God provided Moses under the old covenant, He provides Jesus under the new and better covenant (2 Cor. 3:2-11; Heb. 19:13-15).

The religious authorities despised Jesus during His earthly ministry. They saw Jesus as an impostor, and religious heretic worthy of death. Jesus admitted that these leaders searched the Scriptures. Jesus meant that they studied the Old Testament, and particularly the Books of Moses (Genesis, Exodus, Leviticus, Numbers, and Deuteronomy). Notice what Jesus declares about the Old Testament Scriptures:

> *JOH 5:39 "You search the Scriptures, because you think that in them you have eternal life; and it is these [Scriptures] that bear witness of Me; [brackets mine]*

Jesus is the Exodus story! Moreover, as seen in 2 Corinthians 3:2-11, and Hebrews 19:13-15, believers have a far greater covenant relationship with God than the Hebrews. How much more then is available to believers who are in Christ, Jesus? Believers in-Christ have all they need to overcome any addiction. Specifically, this is a viable program for the homosexually challenged, or person sexually bound or addicted.

Liberation and Deliverance Introduction

The most miraculous story of deliverance occurs in Exodus. The very meaning of the title involves liberation, deliverance, emancipation, and salvation. Given this nation's Christian-Judaic beginnings, both believers and non-believers are acquainted with the man known as the deliverer, Moses.

During December 2000, seven men escaped from a prison in the State of Texas. Eventually, six of the escapees were captured, and one terminated his life. The story of how these men were able to escape outraged residence throughout the state and across the nation. It is amazing and alarming when we are informed about the escape of a dangerous convict. Think of the bewilderment and horror when several convicts escape from a prison in daylight.

While amazing, such experiences pale in comparison to the miraculous and righteous escape recorded in Exodus. Imagine thousands of families with all they own, escaping from the grip of the most powerful empire on earth. Moreover, consider that they overcame centuries of bondage, dehumanization, and socialization without striking a blow, firing a shot, or assassinating a leader. Their sole involvement was their "cry" and preparation for liberation and deliverance (L&D).

Similar to the Bible as a whole, Exodus holds significant and relative meaning for anyone bound and afflicted by man, matter, or man's conditions. This certainly includes any addiction.

Addictions and Addictiveness
A Biblical Perspective
(Part I)

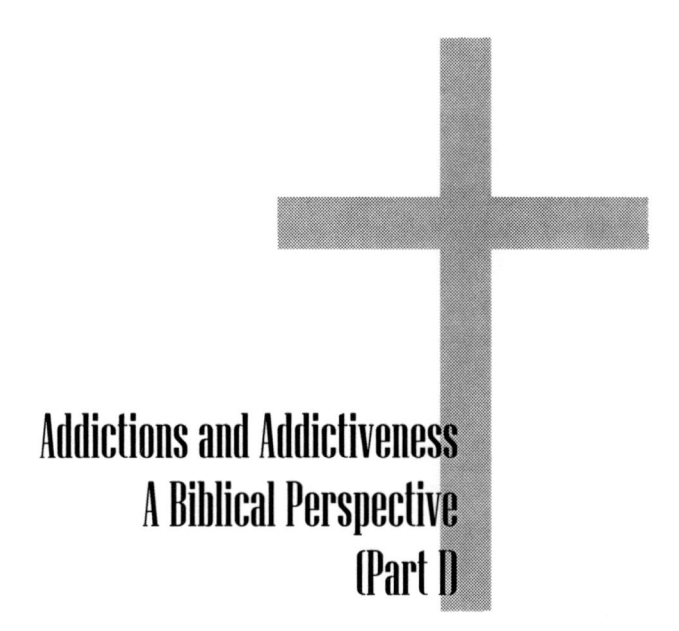

Description of Addiction and Addictiveness

As described in this guide, an addiction is reliance or dependence on a self-destructive behavior, which increases in destructive results while diminishing in pleasure, appreciation, and self-satisfaction. An addiction further affects a person holistically (socially, psychologically, physically, spiritually). Relatives, friends, co-workers, and others usually become aware or hurt by the addict's behavior. The Christ-based Counseling perspective is that an addiction is self-initiated and externally perpetuated. This description is explained later in detail. This program is primarily devoted to the necessary steps to overcome any addiction as described. There are several addictions that are detrimental to believers' ability to fulfill their call or purpose (e.g., prescribed and illegal drugs, sex, eating disorders, excessive exercise, and other similar behaviors). Clearly, some addictions are much more destructive than others. This does not condone any addiction as being more acceptable. However, denial represents such a sophisticated system of rationalization, it is important not to equate an eating disorder with an illicit drug addiction.

The word, habituated is synonymous with the word addiction and its cognates in this counseling guide. Biblically, the word ethos is most often translated, "custom." Customs are a major focus of the New Testament because they often became as important as God's Word among religious leaders (Acts 15:1, 16:21, 21:21). Likewise, habituated-behavior or an addiction has a similar affect on believers. Ethos is also translated, habit, in Hebrews 10:25 (KJV). Some believers made a habit of forsaking the assembly. Nevertheless, the term habituated-believer is used to denote an addiction.

Causes for Addiction and Addictiveness

There is long term research concerning the causes of addiction. Scientists are seeking a genetic cause for every illness known to humanity, and addiction is no different in this regard.

Biblically, believers already have an answer to the scientific quest to find a gene, which predisposes a person to an addiction. A close look at the Biblical record from a CBC perspective reveals an important fact. Sin IS a genetic issue. Sin is a core element of the human gene. However, it is not detectable by scientific instruments. It is a spiritually discerned product of blood (Romans 5:12).

SIN'S GENETIC COMPOSITION CAN ONLY BE DETECTED BY THE MICROSCOPE OF BIBLICAL TRUTH.

Countless believers who suffer with some form of addiction reveal that the first time they participated in the behavior, they chose to participate in spite of the obvious warnings.

Genetic Predisposition: As stated above, some people are more predisposed to certain addictions than other people. However, believers do not face any issue that is not common to man (I Cor. 10:13). Addiction is not new.

The Bible proclaims, "Then the Lord saw that the wickedness of man was great on the earth, and that every intent of the thoughts of his heart was only evil continually" (Gen. 6:5). This verse is the "Genesisial" basis for the description of addiction provided above. Addiction is internally or self initiated, and externally perpetuated. The Lord "saw" the wicked results of man. Moreover, these external results were from every intent of his heart. The key word in the verse is, "continually." The Hebrew word translated, "continually" is comprised of two words yom (day or daily), and kol (whole or all).

It is a matter of record that persons suffering with an addiction as described, possess the center of their world. The addict is the "gravity-core" of his world and those around him. The addict's priority for living becomes the addictive behavior. More specifically, the feeling, euphoria, or other perceived benefit is the goal. The addict will use, manipulate, lie, pander, and abuse anyone or anything to reach the goal.

Genesis 6:5 describes the innate (i.e., in-born), and corporate (i.e., all humanity) nature of addiction, and provides the descriptive term to explain any addiction's duration, "continually." Stated simply, a person actively feeds an addiction externally, by acting upon one's in-born desire. The result is always death [death of dignity, death of relationships, death of mental health, death of spiritual fellowship, and ultimately physical death] (James 1:6).

The addict began by making a choice to indulge the first time. The thinking and decision was made internally, the act was done externally. Thus the description, "self-initiated," and "externally perpetuated."

Some counselees suffering with an addiction disclose that they did not recognize what they were doing when they first began. [See the testimony of Yvette above]. However, this would be the minority, and not a majority of persons suffering with addictions. Moreover, those with protracted addictions [long term] usually claim there were times when they discontinued their behavior. However, they returned to their former behavior. Clearly, persons who returned to their addictive behavior made the choice to return. It is typical for addicts to report they considered the choice for a period before finally capitulating. Whether it is the first time or relapse, the decision was self initiated, and externally perpetuated.

DeGENEration from the Beginning: When Adam sinned, the degeneration process began immediately. Here it is important to restate a Biblical finding from Sex, Sexuality, and the Believer on a homosexual gene. How could there be a homosexual gene?

> The Biblical perspective is that Adam's original sin affected his whole environment, existence, and generations to come (Gen. 3:17-19). It is further understood that God

revealed His principles for living (i.e., commandments, laws, directives), and the primary purpose for these principles was for man to identify objectionable behavior (Rom. 7:7).

The Biblical record further discloses that life of the flesh is in the blood (Lev. 17:11). Therefore, the conditions of sin are passed through bloodlines of all creatures. Paul explains that as the result of Adam's disobedience, sin and its consequences passed from Adam to all humanity. Everyone is incriminated, "even" persons who do not violate principles similar to Adam's violation (Rom. 5:12-14). There are a number of Biblical references demonstrating that sin is through and from birth (Gen. 8:21, Job 15:16, Psa. 51:5, 58:3, John 3:6, Eph. 2:3).

Historically, when God reveals the wickedness of man in Gen. 6:5 as shown previously, the genetic nature of addiction was well established in the human blood stream. David pointedly reveals the genetic aspect of his sinful decision concerning Bathsheba:

PSA 51:4 Against Thee, Thee only, I have sinned, And done what is evil in Thy sight, So that Thou art justified when Thou dost speak, And blameless when Thou dost judge.
PSA 51:5 ¶ Behold, I was brought forth in iniquity, And in sin my mother conceived me.

David's confession in Psalms 51:4 is not followed by an effort to project blame on his parents in Psalms 51:5. He admits his sin personally in 51:4. Psalms 51:5 is simply a statement, which depicts the depth of his and [our] depravity. Both sin and the dynamics, which lead to addiction are the result of our genetic relationship to Adam. Believers need not wait on the research of the "biogenetic" community to discover that sin and thereby addiction is a genetic issue. A CBC description of what caused David to make such a devastating decision will be discussed later.

Comparison between Addictions and the Hebrew's (Pre Deliverance): Perhaps there are those who would view the plight of the Hebrews in Egypt as forced enslavement more than addiction. Those with such a position would argue that the Hebrews were in Egypt in opposition to their will. Therefore, a major difference exists between their liberation and a person desiring to be liberated from a self-initiated and externally perpetuated addiction.

The concerns stated in the preceding argument may appear correct, but the evidence and Biblical truth demonstrates an excellent comparison between the Hebrews' condition and an addiction. There are several relative and important comparisons:

Benefits of Egypt (Survival): The Hebrews introduction into Egypt is recorded in the Book of Genesis. They entered Egypt to maintain their posterity. During the administration of Joseph, Israel's son, the Hebrews entered Egypt to survive, or they would have certainly died (Gen. 41:57-42:2). Upon arrival there, Joseph with the Pharaoh's approval secured the land of Goshen. This was the most fertile and prosperous land in the kingdom (Gen. 47:1-6).

Similarly, people become involved in addictive behavior because of the immediate and obvious benefit. Afterwards, the addictive qualities render the addict helpless. Effectively, the addiction commands a life of its own. It dictates and dominates the addict's life. The Hebrews did not intend to leave Egypt. Well beyond the period of famine, which lasted seven years the Hebrews remained in Egypt. Even after their liberation was secured, they were not crying for liberation from Egypt. They were crying for liberation from the conditions [hardships, forced labor] associated with their relationship, and not crying for liberation from Egypt per se.

Again, this is precisely the case with addictions. The underlying reality is often, the addict's cry is because of the results of the addiction, but not the addiction itself. Briefly stated, the Hebrews loved Egypt, but they despised the bondage. Before a believer can begin the journey to recovery, the believer must come to grips with the sin associated with such behavior. Treating the addiction is not addressing the root cause. The root cause must be addressed, or the person will continue to relapse.

Success in Egypt (Multiplying and success): The Biblical evidence reveals that they assimilated Egyptian culture (Gen. 47:27). Meanwhile, the Hebrews witnessed exponential growth and success. Most addictions give an impression of success, pleasure, satisfaction, and even euphoria in spite of the initial manifestations of problems.

Turn of Events (A new Pharaoh): However, during the course of time a transfer of power occurred. This happened after a number of generations. The Bible proclaims, a Pharaoh arose who did not know Joseph (Exo. 1:8). This does not mean that the Pharaoh did not know about Joseph, historically. It means that with the passage of time and generations, this Pharaoh did not hold the same level of regard for the Hebrews as held by his predecessors. Persons who are struggling with addictions do not experience the same levels of euphoria and satisfaction as experienced when they first began using.

They may or may not accept the reality of the destruction the addiction causes, but the evidence of the destructive effect of their addiction is experienced by those closest to the addict (e.g., spouses, parents, children, friends, employers, etc.). Unfortunately, the addictive quality of their behavior enslaves addicts, and addicts are under the authority of the addiction. Thus, a miraculous intervention is required to liberate and deliver the believer from the addiction.

The Dynamics of Liberation (Part I)

Exodus provides the process of miraculous liberation and deliverance. The Hebrews had to be liberated from Egypt before they could be delivered to the Promised Land. Overcoming an addiction always involves two major categories. If an addict is liberated from addiction, but not delivered to a healthier pattern then returning to Egypt is inevitable.

Cry for Liberation

Well before Moses is called as the deliverer, God heard the cry of his people (Exo. 3:1-7). The "cry" is what moved God to act in behalf of the people. The term "cry" must be discussed and understood. The "cry" in the context of the experience of the Hebrews in Egypt was the result of the depth of their need, the continuous nature of their bondage, and their growing desperation. Therefore, the word cry depicts a deep-seated anguish over a long period under worsening conditions. God responded, "for I have heard the cry of my people." What God hears is the sincere and deep longing in the hearts of his people. What evidence is there of this deep longing? Clearly, the cry or prayers, which are heard by God involve tears, longevity, and consistent pleading (Luke 18:1-8).

Again, we learn from this experience a basic, and yet primary method an addicted person must employ. There must be a cry to the Lord for liberation. This request must be consistent [pray about the same thing], continuous [daily], and over a period of time.

L&D-1, The Habituated-Believer Must Pray Daily For Liberation From Addiction And Deliverance To A New Pattern/Source For Living

Recall, as stated above, the cry is because of the change of events.

God's Purpose

Another truth shown in the Biblical record is that God had a purpose for the liberation and deliverance of the Hebrews. The word is given to Moses, and Moses proclaims to Pharaoh to let God's people go. This liberation is not for the Hebrews. The liberation is for God. This is key to an addict's liberation. One is set free to serve the almighty God. They are set free as a demonstration of God's power in their lives. Moses constantly and consistently gives the reasons for their liberation as follows: Celebrate a feast (5:1), serve Me in the wilderness (7:16), serve Me (8:1), sacrifice to the Lord (8:8), serve Me (8:20), sacrifice to the Lord (8:29), serve Me (9:1), serve Me (9:13), and serve Me (10:3).

Another truth becomes absolutely clear about the origin of the bondage or addiction. Moreover, this truth is that for every godly purpose, there is the objective of our sin nature. Upon departing from Egypt, the Egyptians reconsidered their situation and declared, "What is this we have done, that we have let Israel go from serving us?" Exo. 14:5. Addiction never allows the addict to serve God. Yes, the addict may desire to serve God, but the addiction masters the addict. The addiction is preeminent. The addiction has priority over the family, the addict's on personal well being, and God.

L&D-2 Only God Can Completely Liberate Believers From Habituated-Behavior.

God Calls an Intercessor

It is important to recognize the call of Moses. Moses begins as an insider raised by the Egyptians. He experienced the very best that Egypt had to offer. Egypt was not merely a fledgling nation. Egypt was an empire with great cultural, political, and military influence throughout the ancient world. Many of its artifacts and achievement are still considered some of humanity's most significant achievements. God selected a deliverer who knew the condition because he lived among his brethren (Exo. 2:11). He witnessed the condition, but he did not live under such conditions. Now, this point is particularly important. Often, we believe that the best counselors are persons who have personal experience with the issues they counsel. That is, a person who has experienced addiction is more likely to be an effective counselor of persons suffering with addiction. Persons experiencing marital problems are more likely to be effective counselors of persons encountering marital difficulties. While there is validity to such reasoning, this is not the principle God uses in the case of the Hebrews in bondage. Yes, he certainly uses persons who have made glaring mistakes, as did Moses who murdered an Egyptian.

However, in terms of this specific case, God used Moses who clearly witnessed the depravity of the bondage, but Moses was not under such bondage when God called him.

Similarly and pointedly, Moses was a preview of Jesus. Jesus becomes an insider who experiences our dilemma, but he is an outsider in that he never succumbs to sin. This is what makes an outstanding counselor in the case of addiction. The addicted person needs someone who understands the condition. Someone who has experienced the condition directly or indirectly, but is an outsider who is not under the control or influence of the addiction. This person can proclaim before the world, and in behalf of an addict, "let my brother or sister go."

L&D-3 Habituated-Believers Must Have One Or More Intercessors

God Declares the Time of Liberation

Another principle is that God's liberation is time sensitive. Clearly, a believer's addiction is not a surprise to God. Recall that God told Abraham that his posterity would be in bondage for four hundred years (Gen.15:13). Observe that God made a promise to Abraham. He promised him several things, but most notably that he would be a man of many generations and a chosen people (Gen. 12:2; 13:15-16). However, he also provides information so that Abraham would know that God's promises would not be without challenge. So, Abraham was informed about impending threats to God's promise (Gen. 15:13-14). When everything had been fulfilled that God deemed as needful, he places into motion the liberation and deliverance of the Hebrews. The Hebrews had a spiritual commission to fulfill, and part of that commission required their own homeland. A homeland would distinguish them as God's people. However, when times are fruitful and productive rarely are we focused on God's purpose for our lives. Obviously, the Hebrews were not going to depart Egypt to comply with God's commission if the prosperity they witnessed during Joseph's lifetime and thereafter continued.

It required the passage of time and changing circumstances to reach a level where the Hebrews would cry unto the Lord for liberty.

Here, the CBC, Prodigal Motivation comes into play. The Hebrews depraved condition had to outweigh the benefits experienced in Egypt. This is often referred to as "bottoming-out." However, "bottoming-out" is not the key in a Biblical based L&D program for believers suffering with an addiction. Judas bottomed-out, but Judas did not recover from his obsession with monetary gain. No doubt, he felt guilty and he cast the money away, but that was not the root cause of his problem. The betrayal of Jesus and collection of thirty pieces of silver did not relieve Judas. His natural desires dictated his decisions. Subsequently, he killed himself (Acts 1:16-18).

The addict chooses to begin addictive behavior, but God decides when to liberate the believer. Moreover, when God liberates us from our "Egypts," He does it so that we will never return.

L&D-4 Habituated-Believers Place Their Trust In God's Timing.

God Assaults the Benefactor of the Addiction

Another principle that must be understood by the counselor and counselee alike is that God will assault those persons, things, and systems that benefit from the bondage of His children. This is a Biblical fact. The Biblical record is without exception. Kingdoms, persons and any other entity, which benefit from oppressing God's people, will meet their demise. This is such a serious matter that even when God used other "peoples" to punish His own children, eventually God would destroy the nations He used to punish His own chosen people. It is a principal matter that an enemy of a believer is an enemy of God. Moreover, the enemies of God will be defeated.

L&D-5 God Will Break Anyone Or Anything Supporting A Believer's Habituated Behavior

Relapse Amidst Recovery

Another important concept of this program is to recognize the principle of deception before deliverance, or relapse amidst recovery. Remember, before the Hebrews are liberated it requires a series of plagues and calamities, and these events do not lighten the bondage. Because of these events and the mere request to liberate the Hebrews, the oppression was increased (Exo 5:1-9).

Faith at this point and a faith-filled focus are imperative. The Hebrews were going to be liberated. God had proclaimed it. He did not call the Hebrews to remain in Egypt, and He did not call them to be enslaved to another god who in this case was the Pharaoh.

This is precisely the same principle, which any believer with an addiction can embrace. Notwithstanding what appears to be a worsening situation, God is going to deliver the believer. There is a work in the believer that is to be completed (Ph. 1:6).

Therefore, the addict and significant others who sincerely cry for recovery can expect deceptive events and activities during the recovery process.

Personal Liberation, Interdiction, and Duration

Regardless of the issue, we all want liberation immediately, or at a minimum we desire to see some hopeful signs. This underscores the importance of not choosing to sin, particularly the sin, which leads to an addiction [as defined in this document]. The truth is we only know that when God so decides, the addict will be liberated. Additionally, the addicted believer and those affected must trust the Lord in such matters. As with the Hebrews, God knows the time of liberation. Therefore, instructing believers on interdiction is imperative. How ironic it is that the term, "interdiction" denotes religious prohibition.

Precursor to Liberation: Psalms 51 is classically viewed as David's confession of his sin against God. David's prayer includes the keys to personal liberation. David, describes three focal points, in the first two verses:

> *PSA 51:1 (For the choir director. A Psalm of David, when Nathan the prophet came to him,) (after he had gone in to Bathsheba.) Be gracious to me, O God, according to Thy loving kindness; According to the greatness of Thy compassion blot out my transgressions.*
>
> *PSA 51:2 Wash me thoroughly from my iniquity, And cleanse me from my sin.*
>
> *PSA 51:3 For I know my transgressions, And my sin is ever before me.*

First, David admits a high-minded crime. The term transgression means a premeditated, arrogant, and bodacious violation. His decision to become involved with Bathsheba, and subsequently his plan to have her husband murdered was not by coincidence or serendipitous on either account. These were strategic sins. They required premeditation with appropriate timing, and follow-through.

This is the "addiction threshold." This is the period when the believer is considering the sin, its consequences, and mentally arguing to commit sin. Prior to his sin, there is no doubt that David considered God's commands concerning these issues. The believer must pierce a spiritual hedge to commit a transgression.

Recall, how God boasted about Job. And Satan replied that Job was protected by a hedge (Job 1:1-10), but the classic reference is found in Ecclesiastes. "He that digs a pit shall fall into it, and whoso breaketh a hedge, a serpent shall bite him" (Ecc. 10:8).

L&D-6 Never Pierce A Spiritual Hedge.

David pierced the spiritual walls, reminders and prohibitions, and committed adultery. Subsequently, he murdered Bathsheba's husband. Afterward, Nathan the prophet told David the parable concerning a rich man who had taken the only lamb from a poor man. This allowed David to be an outsider who could judge the acts of the rich man in the parable. David was outraged by the acts of the rich man, and quickly judged the rich man in the story. Responding, Nathan identifies David as the man in the parable, and clearly restates what David thought prior to committing this heinous act.

> *2SA 12:7 Nathan then said to David, "You are the man! Thus says the Lord God of Israel, 'It is I who anointed you king over Israel and it is I who delivered you from the hand of Saul.*

> *2SA 12:8 'I also gave you your master's house and your master's wives into your care, and I gave you the house of Israel and Judah; and if that had been too little, I would have added to you many more things like these!*

Nathan's statements to David are not new revelations. These are precisely the truths David considered just prior to his decision to send for Bathsheba. These are the thoughts that the Spirit brings to our attention when we are contemplating a transgression. There is an ironic comparison between Nathan's words to David, and Joseph's explanation to Potiphar's wife when she attempted to "addict" Joseph:

> *GEN 39:7 And it came about after these events that his master's wife looked with desire at Joseph, and she said, "Lie with me."*

> *GEN 39:8 But he refused and said to his master's wife, "Behold, with me here, my master does not concern himself with anything in the house, and he has put all that he owns in my charge.*

GEN 39:9 "There is no one greater in this house than I, and he has withheld nothing from me except you, because you are his wife. How then could I do this great evil, and sin against God?"

GEN 39:10 And it came about as she spoke to Joseph day after day, that he did not listen to her to lie beside her, or be with her.

Genesis 39:7 reveals that Potiphar's wife desired to have sex with Joseph. Obviously, Joseph could not do anything else for her. He was merely a servant in her husband's household. Notice there is no evidence that she was not an attractive woman. Quite the contrary, Joseph's interdiction is both social and spiritual. First, he gives the social prohibition to such a decision. He considered the trust, honor, and authority Potiphar had given him. The only thing that Potiphar did not give Joseph was his wife. Secondly, there was the spiritual interdiction. Even if Potiphar had not honored Joseph in such a manner, Joseph recognized it would be sin against God almighty to have sex with Potiphar's wife.

During the addiction threshold, Joseph's thinking was clear, persuasive, and determined. Notice Gen. 39:10, Joseph never relents even under the day-to-day pressure she applied. Notice she spoke, but he did not listen to her. This does not mean he did not hear her. He did all that he could not to allow her pleadings to become rooted in his heart. Moreover, he did not allow himself to be with her. Joseph had to stay out of her presence.

L&D-7 Habituated-Believers Must Avoid Addicts Who Encourage Or Influence Habituated-Behavior.

This is spiritual wisdom. The believer must stay out of the presence of people, places, and things that represent the addiction threshold.

There can be no doubt that David had the same thoughts, and same truths to consider as Joseph did. The difference is that Joseph withstood the addiction threshold, but David proceeded.

The David vs. Joseph table shows both of them in the addiction threshold. David fails in the addiction threshold, but Joseph succeeds.

David's Addiction Threshold Failure (2 Samuel 12:7-8)	Joseph's Addiction Threshold Success (Genesis 39: 7-9)
I anointed you over Israel	My master does not concern himself with anything [with me here]
I delivered you from Saul	He put all he owns in my hand
I gave you your master's wives	There's no one greater in this house than I
I gave you Israel and Judah	He's withheld nothing from me
I would add more if that wasn't/isn't enough	[Joseph understood he could have more]
[David proceeds and sends for Bathsheba. 2 Sam 11:3-4]	[Joseph withstands, and stays out of the presence of Potiphar's wife Gen 39:10b.]

Both of these men where called and anointed by God. Both of these men loved God from their youth. Both of these men were heirs of faith and promise. Both were tempted in a similar matter. One of the men withstood, and the other collapsed. This stands as an example, and glaring evidence for every believer who encounters the addiction threshold.

L&D-8 Habituated-Believers Remember The Goodness Of God In The Midst Of The Threshold Battles

Continuing with Psalms 51:2, David does not simply desire to have his transgression blotted out, there is a deeper matter. Secondly, he must address the thing that caused him to trangress. He adds, "Wash me thoroughly from my iniquity, And cleanse me from my sin." Psalms 51:2.

Here, David addresses the thinking process within the addiction threshold. The Hebrew root for the word iniquity means to twist or contort. David twisted the truth, which led to the transgression. This is classic rationalization.

David had to rely on a visceral argument to defeat the great works of God in his life. He had to convince himself that taking another man's wife was warranted. The Bible specifically describes Bathsheba's husband as a Hittite. This fact had some significance in

David's decision.

Hittites were people who occupied Canaan before the Hebrews returned from Egypt. The Hebrews were commanded to destroy the Hittites among others in the land. However, they allowed the Hittites to remain in the land (Exo. 23:23, 28). Generations later David becomes king, and the Hittites are well established in Israel. Clearly, Uriah was an excellent and dedicated officer, but David "marginalized" Uriah. Apparently, David used Uriah's ancestry [in-part] as irrational support for violating his family. The Scripture declares that God was not pleased (2 Sam. 11:27).

David's twisted and perverted thinking is at the very core of his decision to commit adultery. If God does not remove David's ability to twist the truth, justice, and morality, David knows he will repeat the same behavior endlessly.

L&D-9 Habituated-Believers Pray That God Will Straighten Their Twisted Thinking.

How often do addicts speak of circumstances, which led to their behavior? This is particularly the case when we encounter difficult or unpleasant experiences. We desire to do something that will relieve our personal pain, even if it is only for a moment.

Again, Joseph is an excellent example of a person who did not use his circumstances as the purpose for sin.

When Potiphar's wife pleaded with Joseph each day, he could have reasoned that his brothers had betrayed him. Joseph could have acted contrary to the principles taught by his ancestors. After all, he was sold into slavery. He was subject to the whims of his master, or in this case, his master's wife. However, Joseph recognized God's presence in his life in spite of his circumstances. He had a grateful and thankful spirit in the midst of his unfortunate circumstances. He did not use iniquity or twisted thinking to consummate a sexual relationship with Potiphar's wife. He did not twist the truth to support his personal weakness or pleasure.

L&D-10 Habituated-Believers Must Not Use Their Circumstances As An Excuse To Trangress.

Finally, David asked God to forgive him of his sin in general (Psalms 51:2).

Facing the Principal Enemy: A number of Christian counseling models concerning addiction refer to Satan's activity. This program does not credit Satan with personal decisions made by the typical addict. Notice David's prayer in Psalms 51. There is no mention of Satan as the perpetrator of his sin. David conquered many enemies during his lifetime. He defeated lions, bears, Goliath, and countless enemies of the Lord. However, David's greatest foe was his own nature. He rightfully cries out to the Lord, "blot out my transgressions...wash my iniquity...cleanse my sins. Notice the use of the personal possessive, "my."

L&D-11 Habituated-Believers Target Their Own Nature As The Principal Cause For Their Behavior.

The memory factor: Another important aspect of addiction is the lingering or lasting effect of such behavior. Even after the believer is forgiven, and is liberated and delivered from the addictive habit there is often a lingering desire. Yes, the Lord forgives us, and he can remove the very desire for the addictive source. However, many persons who have suffered addiction will tell you that there is a lingering desire that arises on occasion. Moreover, for some, they are continually battling the grip of their addictive behavior. This is what caused David [in part] to say in Psalms 51:3, "my sins are ever before me."

He was forgiven, and there is no record of an endless sense of guilt. He continued with his life. Nevertheless, every time he witnessed an event, which occurred as a result of his personal decision, he was reminded of his sin.

L&D-12 The Residual Effect Of A Transgression Is That Subsequent Addiction Thresholds May Be Indefinite In Duration.

Fortunately, the Lord is greater than our personal desires, and addictive behavior. Given the healing power of God and his intervention, we are able to succeed as Joseph succeeded. Thank God.

Understanding the Threshold: Meanwhile, the L&D process may take the remainder of a person's life. As with all counseling matters, the counselee or addict, and all affected persons desire a quick recovery. Clearly, the addict's faith is imperative. The Hebrews required forty years to conclude a trip that should have taken days (Num. 14:33-34; 32:13).

Sometimes our actions and personal resolve requires years instead of days or months.

Nevertheless, the Lord is primarily interested in one's soul. There can be no doubt that a number of objectives are involved when we are suffering with an addiction resulting from a sinful decision. God intends that we would overcome not only the sin, but that we would also develop resistance to the same or similar sin in the future. There must be substantial character development. Specifically, the addicted believer is to become more like Jesus Christ through the L&D process (Romans 5:1-5; Romans 8:28-29). Rightfully, we want our spouse, child, relative, or friend to return to addiction free living, but God's objective is more eternal in nature. He desires a person who is conformed to the image of His son. Conformation requires victories, successes and progress, but these treasures of life are not possible without disappointment, discouragement, and failure. If a person were to overcome an addiction, but ignore God's eternal purpose then such a recovery is not recovery at all.

Clearly, if a believer does not want to suffer with issues concerning the duration of the liberation process, then interdiction is the key. The believer must be successful within the addiction threshold.

L&D-13 The Ultimate Objective Is That The Habituated-Believer Becomes Conformed To The Image Of Jesus Christ

---

Dynamics of Deliverance (Part III)

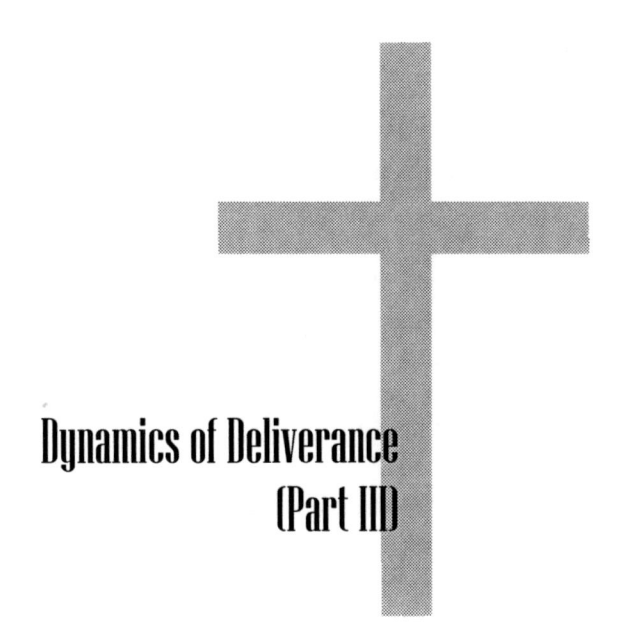

The comparison between addiction and the Hebrews experience after they were liberated continues. Notice, they depart from Egypt on a given day, but the process of being liberated from Egypt required years (Gen. 15:13). Therefore, recovery from a Biblical perspective is completely based on the intervention of God. Yes, there is personal involvement as with all experiences related to the believer's relationship with the Lord.

However, the believer's personal involvement is the result of God's providence upon and around the believer. Often as a result of the circumstances, the believer willfully responds. The circumstances, which led to a will-full response and the response itself, are the result of God's authority.

Biblically, there is no such concept as a person self-correcting one's behavior with bootstraps. Factually, bootstrap mentality is a problem the Lord rebuffs continuously in Scripture (Gen. 15:7; 28:13-15). The addict and persons affected by the addict must understand that it is completely the power, purpose, and providence of God that saves, redeems, rescues, liberates and delivers believers. Certainly, a willing and obedient spirit is required. However, these virtues are the results of God's Word operating in the believer.

L&D-14 God Is Solely Responsible For Believers' Deliverance.

A Period of Praise

Once they witnessed the marvelous liberation by God, the Hebrews established a record of praise (Exodus 15:1-18). Their praises extolled the events surrounding God's final acts against Pharaoh. Early in the delivery process, liberated-believers should write and maintain as a historical record the events leading up to their liberation. It should include a period of celebration. Notice how the women led by Miriam follow the praise with a celebration. Afterwards, the Passover is instituted (Ex 12:11, 21, 43; Lev. 23:5). The very purpose of the Passover was to remember God's intervention in Egypt. This would be passed to every subsequent generation.

L&D-15 Liberated Believers Must Praise God For His Work Of Liberation In Their Lives

Odious Memories

Unfortunately, the Hebrews lived in Egypt for hundreds of years. Once liberated, it was not long before the impact of a new life becomes the overwhelming threat. As time passed, the oppression of Egypt was forgotten, and the pleasures of Egypt became a cherished memory. It is not unusual for liberated believers to forget the sin and hardships associated with their addicted behavior. One would think that after four hundred years of oppression the Hebrews would not dare mention returning to Egypt. Nevertheless, they preferred to return. Likewise, believers who have been liberated from an addiction must remember the goodness and greatness of the God who liberated them. The God who liberates has a plan to deliver.

L&D-16 Liberated Believers Refute Any Pleasure Of Their Habituated Behavior As A Deception, And Look To Ministry Support Opportunities.

Negated Prayers

The celebration was barely over before the Hebrews began complaining about their new life. In addition, this was not merely a subtle complaint. Their complaint included an insult toward the almighty God who liberated them. It is one thing to ask, "what are we going to drink?" But it is clearly another thing to ask such a question and then conclude, "would that we had died by the hands of the Lord in Egypt…when we sat by the pots of meat, when we ate bread to the full" (Exo. 15:23-24; 16:2-3). This is an attitude with grave consequences. First, they were liberated from Egypt, but not delivered to the land of promise. God was not finished. Therefore, their complaining was premature. Their liberation from Egypt was only the beginnings of their experience with God as a liberator. Secondly, their attitude delayed their deliverance. Their attitude represented their faithlessness. Therefore, it virtually negated their prayers. If it had not been for God's covenant with Abraham, it is doubtful that they would have continued at all. Consequently, the unbelieving and complaining generation was not delivered to the Promised Land (Num. 26:64-65; Num. 32:12). Many believers suffer relapse because they were only liberated from their addiction. If a believer is only liberated, and does not continue the program then the believer can expect the obvious.

> **L&D-17 Liberated Believers Can Negate Their Own Prayers with Sarcasm and Impatience, and Postpone or Cancel Their Deliverance**

L&D Programming for Believers Suffering Addictions

Based on the study of God's principles concerning Liberation and Deliverance (L&D), Christ-based Counseling supports the framework for a Biblical L&D program.

Program Activities

- Understanding Addiction, a Biblical Perspective: This section in the counseling guide should be discussed in detail. Counselors should use their creativity and wisdom in developing activities or simply discussing the Biblical perspective of addiction.
- Identifying medical support [if applicable]: If the addiction is substance abuse related, medical programs or support must be discussed. The counselor should determine how long the counselee will be in an L&D program during or after the appropriate medical attention.
- Targeting the Root Cause: A session devoted to understanding the root cause is imperative. This will help the counselee resist any tendency to project fault or blame on anyone else.

- Identifying L&D intercessors: Persons who will pray each day specifically for the counselee must be identified. These should be persons who can be trusted to stay on course. L&D prayers must be offered each day during the program.
- L&D prayer training: This training is for the intercessors. They need to know how important they are in the L&D process. It would be further support if they studied Exodus together with the counselee. A weekly prayer session with the prayer intercessors and counselee combined is recommended. This is best achieved in person at a mutually agreed place and time, but it can also be conducted on the phone or internet.
- Intercessor prayer training, believer: The counselee has to learn the type of prayer required as outlined in the counseling guide. This is not a devotional prayer. This is a cry to the Lord for L&D.
- L&D principles: The counselee needs to learn the principles of Liberation and Deliverance. These should be repeated every session, and they should be committed to memory to the degree possible.
- Threshold training: Counselors must discuss the "addiction threshold" in detail. The counselor should create training scenarios for the counselee to practice. The counselor is encouraged to use the counselee's experiences to create scenarios. Role-playing is an excellent method for training. Train the counselee to bring to memory God's goodness. Train the counselee to identify as a lie any notion that the addicted behavior is pleasurable, etc.
- L&D study (Exodus): The counselee should begin and complete a study of the Book of Exodus during the period. The study should be conducted each day. The study guide is excellent for this purpose.
- Praise Activities: Any progress should be followed by a written praise, which is maintained in the counselee's folder.
- Exploring ministry opportunities (non-leadership): If they are not participating in a Christian related ministry, they should identify one. However, they should not be involved in the leadership of such a ministry during the L&D program.
- Familial support training: Close family members should be briefed concerning the program. Additionally, spouses must be trained on how to support the counselee during the L&D process. The counselee must be informed that the family members will not directly or indirectly support any habituated-behavior.

Program Duration

Depending on the availability of other supports, this program is designed to be anywhere from thirty days to one year. If in-patient detoxification is required and available, thirty days would represent a basic support program after detoxification. Nevertheless, the duration is up to the determination of the counselor of record.

Sessions

Sessions should be held a minimum of once weekly. However, other program constituents should be scheduled to occur daily.

Program Reports

Summary reports should be prepared by the counselor of record on a regular basis. The counselor should prepare a minimum of three reports. One report should be prepared for the initial record. One report should be prepared mid-way through the program. And one report should be prepared at the conclusion of the program. Notes should be taken each session as needed.

Terminating L&D

The program is terminated after the days established at the beginning of the program. The counselor should recommend additional days and activities if necessary. Remember, believers are always in constituent six of Christ-based Counseling. They remain in the process.

L&D Assessment Guide

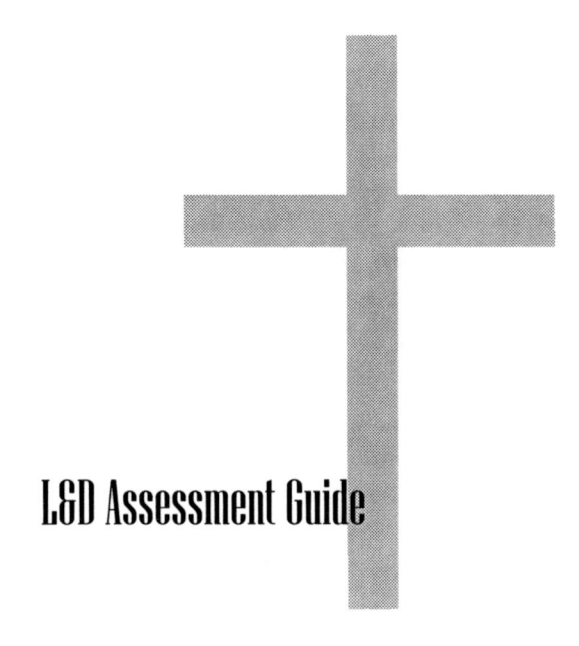

General: This assessment is designed to help the counselor evaluate the counselee's L&D program. The assessment should be conducted during the intake or first counseling sessions, or as soon as it is determined that an addiction is apparent.

Program Activity: A program activity is the component of the L&D program designed to help the counselee learn and apply an L&D principle.

Assessment Concept: The questions in the assessment are specifically related to the first 13 Liberation and Deliverance principles. Once the assessment is completed, the counselor can use the assessment to determine the presence or extent of the counselee's L&D activities. Once a determination is made, the counselor can assist the counselee by making the required arrangements to improve deficient L&D program activities.

Assessment administration: The assessment should be administered periodically to determine the strength of any L&D program activity. This is best administered on a consistent basis such as weekly, bi-weekly, etc.

Understanding the numeric rating: The ratings alone, where

applicable, do not measure how well a person is doing in a certain area. As an example, a person may participate in a behavior once per month. Generally, this is identified as being a good indicator of restraint. However, it does not mean that the practice is more acceptable than something occurring once a week. Committing adultery once per month is a better restraint than a person committing adultery every day. However, committing adultery monthly is much more devastating than a person who is addicted to working numerous hours every day. Therefore, counselors are advised to use discretion. Nevertheless, the higher a rating, the more established the L&D activity is in the counselee's life.

```
Counselee:(Last):_____
(First):_____(MI)____
Address:                                          State:____
Zip:____
Phone:                                Assessment         Date:


Briefly, describe the addiction:

Substance abuse (Drug, alcohol, other) ___ Risk taking ___ Fantasy___
Sex related ___ Gambling ___ Spending ___ Excessive Exercise ___
Work ___ Other ___
```

Answer the following question to the best of your ability:

Directive: L&D-1: Questions 1 through 4 assess the believer's prayer pattern. The counselee must pray daily, and specifically request liberation from addiction.

1. Do you pray?

    Yes [25]
    No [0] (if No go to 5)

2. How often do you take the time, and find a special place to pray?

    Other [1]
    Once monthly [1]

Few times a month [1]
Once weekly [1]
Twice weekly [5]
Three times weekly [10]
Four times weekly [15]
Five times weekly [20]
Everyday [25]

3. When you pray, do you ask the Lord to free you from addiction, or something similar?

   Yes [25]
   No [0] (if No go to 5)

4. When you pray, how often do you ask the Lord to free you from addiction, or something similar?

   Every time I pray [25]
   Often [20]
   Sometimes [10]
   Rarely [1]
   I don't bother, I have to overcome this myself [0]

TOTAL L&D - 1 [_____]

Directive L&D-2: Question 5 assesses whether the counselee fully recognizes that God alone liberates habituated-believers.

5. In your opinion, who is most responsible to liberate you from addiction? 100 pts

TOTAL L&D – 2 [_____]

Directive L&D-3: Questions 6 through 9 assess the support believers' prayer pattern.

6. Is anyone you know praying that you will be freed from addiction?

    Yes [25]
    No [0]

7. Are you sure these persons are praying for you to be freed from addiction?

    Yes [25]
    No [0] (if No go to 10)

8. How often are these other persons praying for you to be freed from addiction?

    Once monthly [1]
    Few times a month [1]
    Once weekly [1]
    Twice weekly [5]
    Three times weekly [10]
    Four times weekly [15]
    Five times weekly [20]
    Everyday [25]
    I am not sure [0]

9. How often do you pray with them to be freed from addiction?

    Everyday [25]
    Often [20]
    Sometimes [10]
    Rarely [5]
    We don't bother, I don't believe praying for something more than once [0]

L&D - 3 TOTAL [_____]

Directive L&D-4: Questions 10 through 15 provide the counselor with general information about the length of the addiction, and the counselee's anxiousness to be liberated. The counselee must learn to trust God's timing. There's no rating for this section.

Understanding the Assessment ■ 189

10. If you could do it, when would you like to be liberated from addiction?

    ☐ Today
    ☐ A week
    ☐ A month
    ☐ A year
    ☐ More than a year

11. If you participated in the addiction activity today, how much time has to pass before you would consider yourself free from the addiction?

    ☐ A day
    ☐ A week
    ☐ A month
    ☐ A year
    ☐ More than a year

12. How old were you when you first participated or exhibited the addictive behavior?

    Age _____

13. How old are you today?

    Age _____

14. Have you ever participated in a recovery program, or attempted yourself to overcome this addiction?

    ☐ Yes
    ☐ No

15. Have you ever relapsed?

    ☐ Yes
    ☐ No

Directive L&D – 5: Questions 16-18 address the system, which supports the believer's addiction. The counselee must understand that the Lord will remove, terminate, or minimize anything or anyone supporting the counselee's addiction. There's no rating for this section.

16. Does anyone or anything "specifically" influence you to participate in this addicted behavior, or helps you participate?

    ☐ Yes
    ☐ No

17. Describe who or what specifically influences you to participate in the addicted behavior?

    ☐ Friend
    ☐ Relative
    ☐ Spouse
    ☐ Other (if Other, briefly explain)

    _____
    _____
    _____
    _____

18. When you feel the urge to participate in addictive behavior, do you ever try to convince yourself not to do it?

    ☐ Yes
    ☐ No (if No go to 20)

Directive L&D – 6: Questions 19-22, assess the presence of the counselee's spiritual hedge, and the degree of restraint. Counselees must be trained to recognize and obey the spiritual hedge.

19. When you feel the urge to participate, how often do you try to convince yourself not to do it?

>   Every time [25]
>   Often [20]
>   Sometimes [10]
>   Rarely [5]
>   I don't bother, I simply do it [0]

20. How often do you participate in this addictive behavior?

>   Daily [0]
>   Weekly [1]
>   Bi Weekly [5]
>   Monthly [10]
>   Beyond monthly [25]

21. Once you make up your mind that you are going to participate in addictive behavior, which best describes how you do it?

>   Every time I do it, it is done away from loved ones [25]
>   Most of the time, secretly from loved ones [10]
>   Sometimes, secretly [5]
>   Everyone around me knows when / how I participate [1]
>   I don't care who knows, I do it whenever I'm ready or feel the urge [0]

22. Once you make up your mind to participate, how often do circumstances, or events occur which indicate that you should not participate in this addicted behavior?

>   ☐ Every time I feel the urge
>   ☐ Often
>   ☐ Sometimes
>   ☐ Rarely
>   ☐ I just go do it

L&D-6 TOTAL [_____]

Directive L&D-7 Questions 23 assesses the believer's exposure to other persons who participate in the same behavior. This should be eliminated, or minimized.

23. How often are you around others who participate in the same addiction you face? (In a non-counseling situation)

>   Daily [0]
>   Weekly [10]
>   Bi Weekly [20]
>   Monthly [40]
>   Beyond monthly [80]

L&D-7 TOTAL [____]

Directive L&D-8: Question 24 assesses the believer's ability to recall God's goodness, and works in his/her life when they are in the "addiction threshold."

24. How often do you recall the goodness God has shown you and His love for you when you are thinking about participating in the addictive behavior?

>   Every time [100]
>   Often [50]
>   Sometimes [25]
>   Rarely [12]
>   Never [0]

L&D-8 TOTAL [____]

Directive L&D-9: Questions 25-26 assess whether the counselee is praying about the thinking pattern. Is the counselee asking God to get to the root cause?

25. When you pray, do you ask God to give you the correct way to think about the addiction you are dealing with?

   Yes [50]
   No [0] (if No go to 27)

26. When you pray, how often do you ask God to correct the way you think about addiction?

   Every time [50]
   Often [30]
   Sometimes [10]
   Rarely [1]
   Never [0]

L&D-9 TOTAL [____]

Directive L&D-10: Questions 27-30 assess the counselee's drive to rationalize the behavior with personal circumstances. The program activity should train the counselee not to rationalize addictive behavior with circumstances.

27. When you feel the urge to participate in this addictive behavior, do you ever think about your circumstances (such as how things are going in your life)?

   Yes [0]
   No [20] (if No go to 30)

28. When you feel the urge to participate in this addictive behavior, how often do you think about your circumstances (such as how things are going in your life)?

   Every time [1]
   Often [5]
   Sometimes [10]
   Rarely [15]
   Never [20]

29. Which are you most likely to think during periods when you consider participating in addictive behavior [concerning circumstances in your life]?

> Generally, things are going very well [20]
> Generally, things are well [15]
> Generally, things are ok [10]
> Generally, things are not well [5]
> It does not really matter to me how things are going [25]

30. Given the following, which is most likely to convince you to participate in the addictive behavior

> The feelings it gives me (any type of mental/emotional) perception [5]
> It reduces the urge [10]
> Gives me something to do [15]
> I don't know [20]
> A combination of the above [10]

L&D - 10 TOTAL [_____]

Directive L&D 11: This assesses who or what the counselee identifies as the cause for the addiction. The answer must be self, or strikingly similar without other contributing factors.

31. If you could identify the number one factor that caused the addictive behavior what would it be? (If you have relapsed, then what caused the relapse)? 100.

L&D - 11 TOTAL [_____]

L&D - 12 is omitted

Directive L&D-13: Question 32, assesses the counselee's purpose for being liberated from addiction. The answer must be to fulfill God's purpose, or something striking similar. If it is placed first assess 99, 2nd equals 66, 3rd equals 33 and if not at all 0.

Understanding the Assessment ▪ 195

32. Give three reasons why you desire to be relieved of this addiction (in order of importance)

   1.

   2.

   3.

L&D-13 TOTAL [____]

Directive L&D-14: This question assesses the counselee's dependence on God to deliver him/her to a new pattern for living

33. Who do you think is solely responsible for "deliverance" to something constructive for you and those around you?

L&D-14 TOTAL [____]

All other L&Ds omitted

TOTAL PROGRAM ASSESSMENT _____ /1100 = _____%

Assessment Scales:

	ACTIVITY ASSESSMENT	TOTAL PROGRAM ASSESSMENT
80-99	Good	Good
60-79	Fair	Fair
40-59	Marginal	Marginal
20-39	Critical	Critical
0-19	Non-existent	

```
Counselee:(Last):_____
(First):_____(MI)____
Address:       _____     State:_____
Zip:_____
Phone:           _____      Assessment      Date:
_____

Briefly describe the addiction:

Substance  abuse  (Drug,  alcohol,  other)____   Risk  taking_____
Fantasy_____
Sex related_____   Gambling_____  Spending____
Excessive Exercise_____   Work_____  Other____
```

Answer the following question to the best of your ability:

1. Do you pray?

    ☐ Yes
    ☐ No (if No go to 5)

2. How often do you take the time, and find a special place to pray?

    ☐ Other
    ☐ Once monthly
    ☐ Few times a month
    ☐ Once weekly
    ☐ Twice weekly
    ☐ Three times weekly
    ☐ Four times weekly
    ☐ Five times weekly
    ☐ Everyday

3. When you pray, do you ask the Lord to free you from addiction, or something similar?

    ☐ Yes
    ☐ No (if No go to 5)

4. When you pray, how often do you ask the Lord to free you from addiction, or something similar?

   ☐ Every time I pray
   ☐ Often
   ☐ Sometimes
   ☐ Rarely
   ☐ I don't bother, I have to overcome this myself

5. In your opinion, who is most responsible to liberate you from the addiction?

6. Is anyone you know praying that you will be freed from addiction?

7. Are you sure these persons are praying for you to be freed from addiction?

   ☐ Yes
   ☐ No (if No go to 10.)

8. How often are these other persons praying for you to be freed from addiction?

   ☐ Once monthly
   ☐ Few times a month
   ☐ Once weekly
   ☐ Twice weekly
   ☐ Three times weekly
   ☐ Four times weekly
   ☐ Five times weekly
   ☐ Everyday
   ☐ I am not sure

9. How often do you pray with them to be freed from addiction?

   ☐ Everyday
   ☐ Often
   ☐ Sometimes
   ☐ Rarely
   ☐ We don't bother, I don't believe in praying for something more than once

10. If you could do it, when would you like to be liberated from addiction?

    ☐ Today
    ☐ A week
    ☐ A month
    ☐ A year
    ☐ More than a year

11. If you participated in the addiction activity today, how much time has to pass before you would consider yourself free from the addiction?

    ☐ A day
    ☐ A week
    ☐ A month
    ☐ A year
    ☐ More than a year

12. How old were you when you first participated or exhibited the addictive behavior?

    Age _____

13. How old are you today?

    Age _____

14. Have you ever participated in a recovery program, or attempted yourself to overcome this addiction?

    ☐ Yes
    ☐ No

15. Have you ever relapsed?

    ☐ Yes
    ☐ No

16. Does anyone or anything "specifically" influence you to participate in this addicted behavior, or helps you participate?

   ☐ Yes
   ☐ No

17. Describe who or what specifically influences you to participate in the addicted behavior?

   ☐ Friend
   ☐ Relative
   ☐ Spouse
   ☐ Other (if Other, briefly explain)

   _____
   _____
   _____

18. When you feel the urge to participate in addictive behavior, do you ever try to convince yourself not to do it?

   ☐ Yes
   ☐ No (if No go to 20)

19. When you feel the urge to participate, how often do you try to convince yourself not to do it?

   ☐ Every time
   ☐ Often
   ☐ Sometimes
   ☐ Rarely
   ☐ I don't bother, I simply do it

20. How often do you participate in this addictive behavior?

   ☐ Daily
   ☐ Weekly
   ☐ Bi Weekly
   ☐ Monthly
   ☐ Beyond monthly

21. Once you make up your mind that you are going to participate in addictive behavior, which best describes how you do it?

    ☐ Every time I do it, it is done away from loved ones
    ☐ Most of the time, secretly from loved ones
    ☐ Sometimes, secretly
    ☐ Everyone around me knows when and how I participate
    ☐ I don't care who knows, I do it whenever I'm ready or feel the urge

22. Once you make up your mind to participate, how often do circumstances, or events occur, which indicate that you should not participate in this addicted behavior?

    ☐ Every time I feel the urge
    ☐ Often
    ☐ Sometimes
    ☐ Rarely
    ☐ I just go do it

23. How often are you around others who participate in the same addiction you face? (In a non-counseling situation)

    ☐ Daily
    ☐ Weekly
    ☐ Bi Weekly
    ☐ Monthly
    ☐ Beyond monthly

24. How often do you recall the goodness God has shown you and His love for you when you are thinking about participating in the addictive behavior?

    ☐ Every time
    ☐ Often
    ☐ Sometimes
    ☐ Rarely
    ☐ Never

25. When you pray, do you ask God to give you the correct way to think about the addiction you are dealing with?

   ☐ Yes
   ☐ No (if No go to 27)

26. When you pray, how often do you ask God to correct the way you think about addiction?

   ☐ Every time
   ☐ Often
   ☐ Sometimes
   ☐ Rarely
   ☐ Never

27. When you feel the urge to participate in this addictive behavior, do you ever think about your circumstances (such as how things are going in your life)?

   ☐ Yes
   ☐ No (if No go to 30)

28. When you feel the urge to participate in this addictive behavior, how often do you think about your circumstances (such as how things are going in your life)?

   ☐ Every time
   ☐ Often
   ☐ Sometimes
   ☐ Rarely
   ☐ Never

29. Which are you most likely to think during periods when you consider participating in addictive behavior [concerning circumstances in your life]?

   ☐ Generally, things are going very well
   ☐ Generally, things are well
   ☐ Generally, things are ok
   ☐ Generally, things are not well
   ☐ It does not really matter to me how things are going

30. Of the following, which is most likely to convince you to participate in the addictive behavior

   ☐ The feelings it gives me (any type of mental/emotional) perception
   ☐ It reduces the urge
   ☐ Gives me something to do
   ☐ I don't know
   ☐ A combination of the above

31. If you could identify the number one factor that caused the addictive behavior what would it be? (If you have relapsed, then what caused the relapse)?

32. Give three reasons why you desire to be relieved of this addiction (in order of importance)

   a.
   b.
   c.

33. Who do you think is solely responsible for "deliverance" to something constructive for you and those around you?

Liberation and Deliverance Follow-up Christ-based Counseling

1. What is one of the most difficult counseling conditions faced by a Christ-based Counselor?

2. What is necessary if you are counseling on a matter other than addiction, and you discover that the counselee has an addiction?

3. Why is it possible to use the same approach to most addictions?

4. Is anyone immune to exhibiting some kind of addictive behavior?

5. Briefly explain what Yvette, and Chuck have in common?

6. In your opinion, which type of addiction receives the most attention

    a. substance abuse
    b. spending (buying)
    c. gambling
    d. sex
    e. work
    f. exercise
    g. Other

7. In your opinion, which seems the most wide-spread?

8. What does the counseling guide state as the most devastating addiction?

9. Discuss whether you believe this is true, and give an example.

10. Briefly describe the seven constituents of Christ-based Counseling.

11. While Moses is known as the deliverer. What claims can we make about Jesus according to the counseling guide?

12. Is the Old Testament, Christ-based? (Please explain your answer, yes or no.)

13. Do believers have a better covenant relationship with God than the Hebrews? (Give supportive scripture)?

Introduction

14. What does Exodus mean?

15. What was the Hebrews sole involvement for their liberation and deliverance?

16. What is L&D?

17. Do you really believe that God has provided a solid basis for liberation and deliverance from addiction through the illustrations of his works in Exodus? (yes or no, please explain)

Addictions and Addictiveness, a Biblical Perspective

18. An addiction is a behavioral habit that can be discontinued at any time.

　　　☐ True
　　　☐ False

19. An addiction is a behavioral habit without any destructive impact.

    ☐ True
    ☐ False

20. An addiction increases in pleasure over time.

    ☐ True
    ☐ False

21. An addiction decreases in pleasure, but requires the same or more participation over time.

    ☐ True
    ☐ False

22. An addiction does not have impact on others.

    ☐ True
    ☐ False

23. An addiction is initiated by someone or something else other than the addicted person.

    ☐ True
    ☐ False

24. An addiction increases in destructive results, while diminishing in pleasure, appreciation, and self satisfaction.

    ☐ True
    ☐ False

25. As opposed to the term addict, what term is used to describe a believer with an addiction?

Causes for Addiction and Addictiveness

26. What are scientists seeking as a cause for addiction?

27. Do believers have an answer to the scientific quest to find a gene, which predisposes a person to an addiction? If so, please briefly explain.

28. Using substance abuse as an example, is this a new problem to mankind? (Use a scripture reference that explains your position)

29. In Genesis 6:5, what does it explain about the intent of mankind's heart?

30. What were the results of man's heart?

31. How often did man consider the intent of his heart?

32. What do "yom" and "kol" mean?

33. What becomes the "addict's" priority for living?

34. What will the "addict" do to reach the goal?

35. According to Gen. 6:5, describe where the root of addiction is?

36. According to Gen. 6;5, describe who is affected?

37. According to Gen. 6:5 how often is the effect apparent?

38. Find James 1:14 in your Bible. Who or what is the primary source of temptation?

39. When a person makes the choice to indulge in addictive behavior, who is responsible?

40. Provide an Old Testament reference and New Testament reference to support your answer to question 40.

Liberation and Deliverance Follow-up Christ-based Counseling ▪ 207

41. Describe what is meant by "self-initiated and externally perpetuated"?

42. Gen. 3:17-19, who or what did Adam's sin affect?

43. What was the primary purpose for God's commandments and laws? Provide a Scriptural reference.

44. Where is the life of the flesh? Provide a Biblical reference.

45. According to Paul, what passed to all mankind as the result of Adam's disobedience?

46. Provide a few Biblical references proving that sin is passed to each person through and from birth?

47. In Psalms 51:4, who does David blame for his adulterous act with Bathsheba?

48. According to David where is the root or origin of such decisions on his behalf?

49. In Psalm 51:5 is David attempting to blame his parents or someone else for his actions?

50. Is David attempting to excuse his actions?

51. How does discussing the sin content of human blood help counselors and counselees to understand the origin of addiction?

52. What two entities does the guide compare as having similar experiences?

53. Why did the Hebrews enter Egypt?

54. Who decided where the Hebrews would live in Goshen?

55. Was there anything unique about Goshen? Explain.

56. Were there benefits for the Hebrews to live in Egypt?

57. Were the Hebrews crying to leave Egypt, or to be freed from the oppression of Egypt.

58. Do persons who are addicted participate because of the benefits of such an addiction?

59. Do persons who battle addiction desire to be freed because of the addiction itself, or the impact?

60. What must an addicted person come to grips with before lasting recovery is possible?

61. Where the Hebrews successful in Egypt?

62. Do most addictions give an impression of success?

63. When a Pharaoh arose that did not know Joseph, what likely does this mean?

64. Do persons struggling with addictions sense the same levels of euphoria and satisfaction as when they first began such behavior?

65. When persons suffering with an addiction do not accept the destructive effect of such behavior, give examples of persons most likely to recognize the impact first?

66. Who or what is the authority in the addict's life?

67. What is required to liberate and deliver an addicted person?

The Dynamics of Liberation

68. What Book in the Bible provides the process of miraculous liberation and deliverance?

69. What are the two major categories required to overcome an addiction?

Liberation and Deliverance Follow-up Christ-based Counseling ▪ 209

70. If a person with an addiction is liberated from the behavior, but not delivered to a more healthy pattern and practice, what is likely?

71. Did God hear the cry of the Hebrews before he called Moses?

72. What moved God to act in their behalf?

73. Give three characteristics describing the Hebrews cry?

74. Read Luke 18:1-8. Why does the woman in Jesus' parable continue to plead with the unjust judge?

75. What is the result of the woman's plea?

76. What is Jesus teaching us about our prayer/petitions before our just God?

77. So, what is necessary for the habituated-believer to be liberated?

78. What are the three characteristics of the request for liberation?

79. What is the first L&D principle?

80. Who had a purpose for the liberation and deliverance of the Hebrews?

81. Provide an example of at least two reasons why Pharaoh must release the Hebrews according to Moses?

82. What is the Biblical purpose to desire liberation from an addiction?

83. Is an addiction designed to allow the believer to serve God?

84. What does the addiction have authority over?

85. What does L&D-2 state?

86. Was Moses raised with the benefits of Egypt?

87. Egypt was a weak nation.

    ☐ True
    ☐ False

88. Egypt was a world empire.

    ☐ True
    ☐ False

89. Moses was a Hebrew himself.

    ☐ True
    ☐ False

90. Moses witnessed the oppression of the Hebrews, and he also was oppressed.

    ☐ True
    ☐ False

91. Moses lived in the household of the Pharaoh.

    ☐ True
    ☐ False

92. The Lord caused Moses to rebel against Egypt with military power.

    ☐ True
    ☐ False

93. Moses was a preview of whom?

94. Explain how Jesus is an insider and outsider to believer's experience.

95. Concerning relationship to the habituated-believer's condition, what does the believer need?

Liberation and Deliverance Follow-up Christ-based Counseling ▪ 211

96. Explain L&D-3

97. Is a believer's addiction or relapse a surprise to God?

98. Years before the bondage of the Hebrews, what did God tell Abraham?

99. Did God make a promise to Abraham?

100. Briefly explain the promise concerning Abraham's offspring.

101. Was God's promise to Abraham without challenges?

102. Why did the Hebrews need their own homeland?

103. What is likely to be our response to God when times are good?

104. What was required to motivate the Hebrews to cry unto the Lord?

105. Is "bottoming-out" a key in a Biblical based L&D program?

106. Who serves as an example to demonstrate that simply "bottoming-out" may be completely meaningless?

107. Who chooses when to begin addictive behavior?

108. Given that the habituated-believer is crying to the Lord for liberation daily, who decides when to liberate the believer?

109. Explain L&D-4

110. Why wouldn't you want to be a person who contributes to the addiction of a believer?

111. Eventually, what will happen to kingdoms, persons, and other entities, which benefit from addicting a habituated-believer?

112. Explain L&D-5

113. What did God unleash on Pharaoh to convince him to release God's people?

114. When he learned of God's desire to liberate the Hebrews, how did the Pharaoh respond toward the Hebrews?

115. Is it true, Biblically, that when a person desires to be liberated, conditions could become worse before liberation is attained?

116. In spite of their worsening circumstances, what must the habituated-believer trust that God is going to do?

117. What promise can the habituated-believer cling to which proves that he/she will complete his/her work for the Lord? Provide the Biblical reference.

118. How soon do habituated-believers desire to be liberated?

119. Why is it so important not to commit a sin, which leads to an addiction?

120. What does "interdiction" mean as described in this guide?

121. Who provides an excellent example of keys to personal liberation?

122. What does David admit first in Psalms 51:1?

123. What is a transgression?

124. Explain the "addiction threshold."

125. Did David consider God's commands concerning adultery before he committed adultery?

126. What must be pierced to commit a transgression?

127. When God boasted on Job, what did Satan say was protecting Job?

Liberation and Deliverance Follow-up Christ-based Counseling ▪ 213

128. What does Ecc. 10:8 warn about breaking a hedge?

129. What does L&D-6 state?

130. Read 2 Sam. 11:26-27. When David committed adultery with Bathsheba, and had her husband murdered, did he continue to have sex with her?

131. Did David think that he covered his sin?

132. Who was the prophet that revealed David's sin?

133. Give an example of the things God did for David that should have prevented him from losing in the addiction threshold, concerning Bathsheba.

134. Are Nathan's statements about what God has done for David new revelations?

135. What would lead you to believe that David had these thoughts before he committed the sin?

136. Who attempted to get Joseph to participate in a sin, which would lead to an addiction?

137. What did this person want Joseph to do?

138. What's Joseph's social interdiction to accepting the offer?

139. What's Joseph's spiritual interdiction to accepting the offer?

140. How often was Joseph pressured to indulge himself sexually?

141. Did Joseph listen to the sexual offers?

142. Did Joseph hear the sexual offers?

143. What did Joseph do to win the daily addiction threshold battles?

144. What does L&D-7 state?

214 ▪ Christ-based Counseling Handbook

145. What is the difference between Joseph and David within the addiction threshold?

146. What specifically does Joseph recall to memory when he was in the midst of the threshold?

147. David was called and anointed.

    ☐ True
    ☐ False

148. Joseph was not called and anointed.

    ☐ True
    ☐ False

149. Only one of them was an heir of faith and promise.

    ☐ True
    ☐ False

150. Both of them were tempted sexually.

    ☐ True
    ☐ False

151. Both of them failed in the addiction threshold.

    ☐ True
    ☐ False

152. What do believers remember in the midst of the threshold battles?

153. After his transgressions are blotted out, what else does David desire?

154. What does iniquity mean?

Liberation and Deliverance Follow-up Christ-based Counseling ■ 215

155. What did David have to rely on to defeat the great works of God in his life?

156. Did David have to convince himself that taking another man's wife was somehow warranted?

157. When David inquired about Bathsheba, what did the writer specify about Bathsheba's husband?

158. Who were the Hittites?

159. Is Uriah's nationality an additional reason for David to draw closer to committing adultery with his wife?

160. What will happen if God does not "wash" David's ability to twist or rationalize the truth?

161. Briefly state L&D-9?

162. Do habituated-believers often think about their circumstances to justify their behavior?

163. Who is an example of a person who resisted and won the "threshold battles" each day?

164. What circumstances could this person use to support accepting the offers of Potiphar's wife?

165. What or who did he recognize in his life in spite of his circumstances?

166. What kind of attitude did he have in the midst of his unfortunate circumstances?

167. Explain L&D-10

168. After asking God to blot out his transgressions and wash his iniquities, what thirdly does David ask?

216 ■ Christ-based Counseling Handbook

169. Who is not credited with the decisions made by the habituated believer in the addiction threshold?

170. Does David mention Satan as the person responsible for his transgressions?

171. Does David mention Satan as the person responsible for his iniquity?

172. Does David mention Satan as the person responsible for his sins?

173. Who or what was David's greatest foe?

174. Read Romans Chapter 7. Given David's confessions in Psalms 51 and Paul's writings in Romans Chapter 7, who or what must the habituated learn to overcome?

175. The key to overcoming the principal enemy for a habituated-believer is to ask the Lord daily to BWC. What is BWC?

176. Briefly explain L&D-11.

177. What is often the result of an addiction after the habituated-believer has overcome the practice or behavior?

178. What do habituated-believers often express after they have overcome the habituated practice or behavior?

179. What did David say, or how did he refer to this condition?

180. Did David make his statement out of guilt, or the constant reminder of results he caused?

181. Explain L&D-12

182. Who serves as an example that we can be victorious in each threshold battle whether before an addiction is conceived or afterward?

183. Who enables such an ability within us?

184. How long can the L&D process take?

185. What would you state to a habituated-believer's question about how long it will take to overcome the addiction?

186. What Biblical example would you give?

187. What is God's primary interest?

188. What does God intend?

189. What or who is the believer to become more like through the L&D process?

190. What is often a spouse, child, or relative's desire for the habituated-believer?

191. What is God's desire?

192. What does conformation require?

193. What is the irony of a person who recovers, but ignores God's eternal purpose?

194. What is key if a believer does not desire to suffer with issues such as the duration of the liberation process?

195. Briefly discuss L&D-13.

Dynamics of Deliverance

196. The Hebrews were liberated from Egypt on a given day. Did it take a day to liberate the Hebrews? Explain.

197. Who must intervene for a habituated-believer to be liberated?

198. Is there personal involvement by the believer?

199. Who motivates the believer's response or participation?

200. What often causes the believer to respond willfully?

201. Can a habituated-believer use the bootstrap mentality?

202. Who has the power and provides the way for the habituated believer to be delivered?

203. Briefly discuss L&D 14.

204. Once God liberated the Hebrews, what was one of their first acts?

205. When a habituated-believer is liberated, what exercise should the believer practice?

206. What else did the Hebrews institute?

207. Briefly explain L&D 15

208. Once liberated, what becomes the overwhelming threat?

209. As time passes, what might a habituated-believer forget, and what becomes a cherished memory?

210. What must believers remember who have been liberated from addictive behavior?

211. Briefly explain L&D-16

212. What was the object of the Hebrews' complaint initially?

213. Was their complaint subtle? Explain.

214. What did their attitude do?

215. What caused God to continue with the Hebrews?

216. What happened to the unbelieving and complaining generation?

217. Why do many habituated-believers suffer relapse?

218. Briefly explain L&D -17.

219. The following is a series of counseling scenarios. Outline an L&D program for each one.

    You are counseling a couple, and the husband is constantly promiscuous in spite of his personal desire to do otherwise. Outline an L&D program for him.

    You are counseling a couple, and the wife has a spending habit that she cannot control. Outline an L&D program for her.

    You are counseling a young-adult who has a substance abuse addiction. Outline an L&D program for her.

Note: A complete study of Exodus is recommended. The course is available on the internet at Christbasedcounseling.org.

Joy Therapy

Joy Therapy
Overcoming Depression
A Christ-based Counseling Approach

Author and Empowerment: Jesus Christ

Doctrinal Writing: Paul of Tarsus the Apostle

Counseling Design: Dr. Steven DavidSon

Objective: Believers will learn the steps to overcome depression.

Purpose: The purpose of providing the approach is NOT for believers to overcome depression and indulge in personal and self-oriented desires. The purpose for Christ-based Counseling is for believers to accomplish the will of the Lord in their lives. Therefore, any therapy with a Christ-based purpose is to encourage the person to pursue Christian virtues.

Target Persons: This approach is for believers who seek a Christ-based alternative.

Caution: Believers who are known to have psychotic or catatonic episodes when they abstain from the use of prescribed drugs must continue drug therapy. And in any case, persons using prescribed drugs must seek the support and approval of their physician.

Introduction

Second most frequent counseling issue: I have found in my counseling ministry covering more than eighteen years, mood disorders (i.e., Depression, Bipolar, Seasonal, etc.) represent the second highest counseling issue faced by believers.

Christ-based Counseling and Historic Truths: Excluding manifestations of a chemical imbalance, believers who KNOW what they have in Jesus Christ do not suffer from circumstantial depression. Depression based on a believer's circumstances is rooted in Biblical or spiritual immaturity. Emphatically, believers who intimately and experientially know the reality of Christ in their lives DO NOT suffer from depression as technically defined. They may experience grief, sadness, sorrow, and discouragement, but not depression. Moreover, contemporary humanity did not suddenly "catch" depression. A condition has merely been defined, which always existed. Whatever the condition, the Lord provides healing support for His people to accomplish their purpose in Him.

Technical Description of Depression (abbreviated): DSM-IV is the clinician's guide to diagnoses of mood disorders. Briefly stated, DSM-IV guides the clinician to look for a combination of five or more of the following: fatigue, slowed speech, agitation, guilt, low self-esteem, suicidal, death wish, obsessions, compulsions, crying spells, or phobias. Other symptoms may include loss of interests, eating disorders and sleeping disorders. It further states, "patients may admit feelings of hopelessness, helplessness and worthlessness." **Note: This is not a personal diagnosis, but this is here to provide a description of likely symptoms according to the guide.**

Whether stated or not by the patient, these three feelings are the underlying basis of most mood disorders.

Biblical Truth: Regardless of FEELINGS, believers ARE NOT hopeless, helpless or worthless.

Biblical and Therapeutic Design: While Biblical content

throughout Scripture supports the Biblical and Counseling truths stated above, all of the guidance required in this therapy are stated chronologically in the book of Philippians. This is designed so that any believer can follow Paul's advice and inferences as presented in this therapy. Paul is the writer of Philippians.

Joy Defined

Cognates or Family Words: Joy, rejoice, charisma, grace, are all from the same root.

DavidSon's Definition of Joy: A believer's internal assurance of one's eternal destination (joy of faith) Phil. 1:26.

Source of Christian Joy: JOY is a bi-product of salvation. When a person is born again, the believer has the assurance that one's eternal destination is secured. Understand, these are the persons who are "good" ground hearers of God's Word. Jesus says, these persons hold on to His Word (Mark 4:15-20; Luke 8:11-15). The good ground hearer, by-definition, is eternally secure. The other three hearers who all look like believers may not be eternally secure, but the "good" ground hearer is SECURE. Therefore, the question is, whether the counselee has embraced God's Word as the empowerment for daily living and eternal life. The good ground hearer represents the standard of belief necessary to live a productive and victorious Christian life.

Occurrences of Joy in Philippians: Arguably, Philippians is the champion of Biblical books on the topic of joy and rejoicing. Each occurrence is restated for your consideration:

> *PHI 1:25 And having this confidence, I know that I shall abide and continue with you all for your furtherance and **joy** of faith;*
>
> *PHI 1:26 That your **rejoicing** may be more abundant in Jesus Christ for me by my coming to you again.*
>
> *PHI 2:2 Fulfil ye my **joy**, that ye be likeminded, having the same love, being of one accord, of one mind.*
>
> *PHI 2:16 Holding forth the word of life; that I may **rejoice** in the day of Christ, that I have not run in vain, neither laboured in vain.*

> *PHI 2:17 Yea, and if I be offered upon the sacrifice and service of your faith, I **joy**, and **rejoice** with you all.*
>
> *PHI 2:18 For the same cause also do ye **joy**, and **rejoice** with me.*
>
> *PHI 3:1 Finally, my brethren, **rejoice** in the Lord. To write the same things to you, to me indeed is not grievous, but for you it is safe.*
>
> *PHI 4:1 Therefore, my brethren, dearly beloved and longed for, my **joy** and crown, so stand fast in the Lord, my dearly beloved.*
>
> *PHI 4:4 **Rejoice** in the Lord alway: and again I say, **Rejoice**.*
>
> *PHI 4:10 But I **rejoiced** in the Lord greatly, that now at the last your care of me hath flourished again; wherein ye were also careful, but ye lacked opportunity.*

The Test of Joy: You cannot KNOW that you have the joy of faith, or Christian joy until you encounter sorrow. It is amazing to consider that the person who speaks and expresses joy so fervently above is "unhappy" and sorrow-filled concerning his personal circumstances. The Biblical evidence makes it clear that Paul saw his circumstances in prison as sad and afflicted (Paul's sad and sorrow-filled circumstances):

> *PHI 1:12 ¶ Now I want you to know, brethren, that my circumstances have turned out for the greater progress of the gospel,*
>
> *PHI 1:13 so that my imprisonment in the cause of Christ has become well known throughout the whole praetorian guard and to everyone else,*
>
> *PHI 2:27 For indeed he was sick nigh unto death: but God had mercy on him; and not on him only, but on me also, lest I should have **sorrow** upon **sorrow**.*

*PHI 3:8 Yea doubtless, and I count all things but loss for the excellency of the knowledge of Christ Jesus my Lord: for whom I have **suffered** the **loss** of **all things**, and do count them but dung, that I may win Christ,*

*PHI 4:14 Nevertheless, you have done well to share with me in my **affliction**.*

How could a man do this? Here is a man who lost everything he had, and was in prison for preaching Jesus Christ. How could he express joy, and encourage those who were free to rejoice in the Lord always?

Joy Therapy

<u>The Battle for Your Mind:</u> Preachers, teachers and others constantly speak of the necessity to read and study God's Word. Each believer must have the mental training, and spiritual preparation to win the day-to-day mental battles. Believers need to know and see their circumstances from a Biblical perspective. Paul knew how to live through difficult and tragic circumstances without mood altering substances. We have the same principles available to us, and our circumstances are probably not as deplorable and sad as Paul's. Here are seven steps to overcome mood disorders. Place these on your walls, or anywhere they can be helpful. Repeat or practice these when any of the symptoms stated above occur. Persons who are not suffering with a mood disorder should learn and practice these for preventive reasons.

<u>Done Deal Mentality</u> (Know that the Lord will finish His work in you): The believer who is in an intimate relationship with Christ is assured that Jesus will complete the work He began in the believer. Paul knew and he states:

*PHI 1:6 For I am **confident** of this very thing, that He who began a good work in you will perfect it until the day of Christ Jesus.*

Regardless of feelings, the believer has a unique purpose in God's plan, and Jesus is going to fulfill that purpose in YOU!

Winner's Mentality: (The Lord made it possible, that come what may, WE WIN): Believers need to anticipate victory over every challenge. Winners expect to win. However, the key here is we do not win because of our own strength. We win because of what God has done through Christ, Jesus. Paul has such a winning mentality that whether he lived or died, he would WIN. He states,

> PHI 1:21 For to me, to live is Christ, and to die is gain.

Physical death results in the greatest victory of all for believers. Yes, we succumb to some battles, but we always know that we have won, and we are winning. We shall win the war. If I live, I'll live for Christ and if I die, "precious" in the sight of the Lord is the death of his saints (Psa. 116:15).

Help Somebody Mentality (Help with the issues of others): I have discovered that often believers who suffer most from mood disorders are not involved in any helping ministry. They are almost always looking for someone to help them. Paul clearly demonstrates from prison that joy will cause us to edify and encourage others. Minimally, believers should be able to pray for others. Paul states:

> PHI 2:2 Fulfil ye my joy, that ye be **likeminded**, having the same love, being of one accord, of one **mind**.

> PHI 2:3 Let nothing be done through strife or vainglory; but in lowliness of **mind** let each esteem other better than themselves.

> PHI 2:5 Let this **mind** be in you, which was also in Christ Jesus:

> PHI 2:6 who, although He existed in the form of God, did not regard equality with God a thing to be grasped,

> PHI 2:7 but emptied Himself, taking the form of a bond-servant, and being made in the likeness of men.

> PHI 2:8 And being found in appearance as a man, He humbled Himself by becoming obedient to the point of death, even death on a cross.

Cited as the example of service in the midst of pain and suffering, Jesus humbled himself and died for us.

<u>Finish-line Mentality</u> (If it hurts don't look back. Keep your eye on the spiritual PRIZE ahead): While it is popular, and psychologically preferred to constantly recall and repeat unfortunate abuses and maltreatment, the believer does not depend on the "mystery or magic" of recalling and rehashing these awful experiences. Biblically speaking, we all come from horrid, sin-filled and degenerated circumstances (Psa. 51:5, Rom. 3:23). Certainly, many believers have experienced dire and depraved circumstances (e.g., rape, incest, molestation, etc.). These are experiences where "closure" may not exist. And closure is not necessary for the believer. Thank God, Jesus Christ brings closure to any condition. The spiritual principle is to concentrate on our "new" creation beginnings (2 Cor. 5:17). Paul continues:

PHI 3:13 Brethren, I count not myself to have apprehended: but this one thing I do, <u>forgetting</u> those things which are behind, and reaching forth unto those things which are before,

PHI 3:14 I press toward the mark for the prize of the high calling of God in Christ Jesus.

*PHI 3:15 Let us therefore, as many as be perfect, be thus **<u>minded:</u>** and if in any thing ye be otherwise **<u>minded,</u>** God shall reveal even this unto you.*

Our most significant concern should be our spiritual purpose, and not successes, life's possessions, or personal circumstances.

<u>Don't Worry Mentality</u> (Do not anticipate that the worse is going to happen): Consistent with Jesus guiding principles for us not to worry (Matt. 6:32-33), Paul provides an outstanding Word-therapy. He not only tell us what NOT-TOO-DO, he explains WHAT-TOO-DO. Paul instructs as follows:

PHI 4:6 Be careful for nothing [don't worry]; but in every thing by prayer and supplication with thanksgiving let your requests be made known unto God.

> *PHI 4:7 And the peace of God, which passeth all understanding, shall keep your hearts and **minds** through Christ Jesus.*
>
> *PHI 4:8 ¶ Finally, brethren, whatever is true, whatever is honorable, whatever is right, whatever is pure, whatever is lovely, whatever is of good repute, if there is any excellence and if anything worthy of praise, let your **mind** dwell on these things.*

Again, regardless of how one feels, the believer must continue with determination. If the believer does what Paul has instructed, the believer will discover an indescribable peace—in the midst of personal difficulty. Be sure to prepare a list of things true, honorable, right, pure, lovely, good repute, excellence, praise worthy, AND let your MIND dwell or live on these things.

<u>Contentment Mentality</u> (Stop struggling for circumstances you THINK you want): Often persons who suffer with mood disorders are constantly striving or struggling for different circumstances in some area of their lives. We must believe that God is using our current circumstances to build Christian character, and shape us into the image of His son (Romans 5:1-8; Romans 8:28-29). He will change our circumstances when He has completed the use of that particular situation. This does not mean a believer should not desire different circumstances. The believer does not have to strain and struggle. The Lord will change the believer, or the believer's circumstances when He has accomplished His will. Paul learned the following:

> *PHI 4:11 Not that I speak from want; for I have **learned** to be content in whatever circumstances I am.*
>
> *PHI 4:12 I **know how** to get along with humble means, and I also **know how** to live in prosperity; in any and every circumstance I have **learned** the secret of being filled and going hungry, both of having abundance and suffering need.*

Paul has learned the secret of contentment and being filled or hungry. Here's the SECRET: (PHI 4:13 I can do all things through Him who strengthens me).

<u>All You Need Mentality</u> (Understand that God will provide ALL you need): Believers who know intimately what they have in Jesus are CONVINCED that God will provide whatever the need may be. Paul who was not able to repay the Philippians for their gifts reminds them of the one who will provide. He states:

> *PHI 4:19 And my God shall supply all your needs according to His riches in glory in Christ Jesus.*

Now, believers who employ, embrace, concentrate and repetitively practice the seven steps of Joy Therapy will know JOY AND never experience depression as defined. Joy Therapy for circumstantial depression is summarized as follows:

1. Done-Deal Mentality (Know that the Lord will finish his work in you) Phil. 1:6.
2. Winner's Mentality: (The Lord made it possible, WE WIN) Phil. 1:21.
3. Help Somebody Mentality (Help with the issues of others) Phil. 2:2-5.
4. Finish-line Mentality (If it hurts don't look back. Keep your eye on the spiritual PRIZE ahead) Phil. 3:13-15.
5. Don't Worry Mentality (Do not anticipate that the worse is going to happen) Phil. 4:6-8.
6. Contentment Mentality (Stop struggling for circumstances you THINK you want) Phil. 4:11-13.
7. All You Need Mentality (Understand that God will provide ALL you need) Phil. 4:19.

"The joy I have, the world did not give it to me, and the world cannot take it away." (Final quote, author unknown).

College of Professional Christian Studies (Global)
Departments of Biblical Studies and Christ-based Counseling

COURSE: Joy Therapy for Mood Disorders

Practicum Requirement:

Course Literature: Read Joy Therapy

Pre-requisites (if any): Also, must complete Study in Philippians course for credit.

Understanding the Course Design

Candidates use the literature to respond to questions

Answers: Answers must be given in complete sentences.

1. What is the objective of this approach?

    1a. What is the stated purpose of using this approach to overcome forms of depression?

1b. Briefly explain the caution that is given to counselees?

2. Describe the Christ-based Counseling Truth of this therapy?

3. What are the two exceptions, which demonstrate why believers suffer with depression (see Counseling Truth)?

4. Name several of the indicators clinicians use to diagnose depression.

   4a. Whether stated or implied, what are the three feelings underlying most mood disorders?

   4b. State the Biblical Truth?

   4c. Where would a believer find all of the texts in this therapy?

5. What are some of the words in the same family group as the word, joy?

6. According to Dr. DavidSon, what is joy?

7. Given DavidSon's description, what or who is the source of our joy?

8. Read Mark 4:15-20 and Luke 8:11-15. Answer the following: Who tells the parable in the texts?

9. How many types of hearers are there?

10. Give the names of the four types of hearers?

11. Explain what happens to the wayside or first hearer?

12. Explain what happens to the stony ground, or second hearer?

13. Explain what happens to the third or thorns and thistle hearer?

14. Explain the characteristics of the fourth or good ground hearer?

15. According to the therapy, what is the question concerning the counselee?

16. How often does the words joy, rejoice, or rejoicing occur in Philippians?

17. Provide an example of some of the verses?

18. What must occur before a person can really experience or know joy?

19. What is amazing about the person who gave so many expressions of joy in the Book of Philippians?

20. Was Paul happy or sorrow-filled concerning his circumstances? Briefly explain?

21. Where was Paul located?

22. Who witnessed Paul's imprisonment for the cause of Christ within the prison?

23. What do most ministers encourage others to do concerning God's Word?

24. What does each believer need mentally?

25. What do believers need to do concerning their circumstances?

26. What did Paul know how to do without mood altering substances?

27. Are the same principles and power, which Paul depended on available to us?

28. Will most of us face circumstances as deplorable as Paul's (e.g., condition, unjust, maltreatment, etc.)?

29. How many "Mentalities" or principles are there for overcoming circumstance-based mood disorders?

30. Where might a person post these principles as a reminder?

31. Why should persons who are not suffering with such difficulties learn these principles?

32. What is the Done Deal Mentality (DDM)?

33. What type of relationship must the believer have with Christ?

34. What verse in Philippians supports the DDM?

35. What do we mean by "Winners Mentality" (WM)?

36. What text in Philippians support Winner's Mentality?

37. What does death lead to concerning believers (WM)?

38. What is "precious" in the sight of the Lord?

39. Describe Help Somebody Mentality (HSM)?

40. What does Paul clearly demonstrate from prison that joy will do?

41. Which verses support this principle, and what part of our body does Paul target?

42. Explain Finish Line Mentality (FLM)?

43. Biblically speaking and regardless of success, prestige, status or wealth, what is our true condition, AND what is more important to concentrate on?

44. What verses in Philippians 3 supports (FLM)?

45. According to FLM, what is our most significant goal and purpose?

46. Explain Don't Worry Mentality (DWM)?

47. In detail, explain what we are to do in vss 6-8

48. Describe the Contentment Mentality (CM)?

49. Did Paul always know how to be content, AND what did he know what to do with AND without?

50. Who is the secret, which Paul learned, AND what is Paul able to do with this Secret?

51. Describe All You Need Mentality (AYNM)?

52. What are believers who have an intimate relationship with Jesus convinced?

53. What scripture supports (AYNM)?

54. What is necessary NOW for believers who want to know JOY and never experience circumstance-based depression?

Appendix

Marriage Enhancement Program

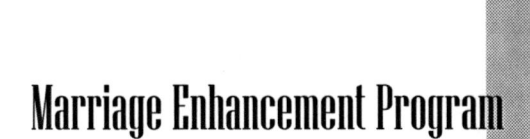

Christ-based Counseling Mental Truths

"My mind must be transformed" (Romans 12:2)
"My thoughts must be guarded" (Ephesians 6:16)

And

REMEMBER, RECALL, AND RESTATE:

*"No matter how tragic, excellent, or endless my experience
I'm being conformed to the image of Jesus Christ"
(Romans 8:28-29)*

Christ-base Counseling
Marriage Enhancement Program

Transforming Rebels and Tyrants

to
Wives and Husbands

It is not news for anyone concerning the incredible rate of divorce in our nation. As a Christ-based counselor, it is clear the Christian community is as affected by the assault on the marital union as any other demographic of our society.

Obviously, we seek and search for an answer. Books are written in volumes on how to maintain healthy relationships. There are seminars, workshops, and degree programs designed to embellish marital ties and family relationships.

I am certainly no different in this regard. Spending enormous hours investing in family, I am gratified by the results I have witnessed in the Christ-based counseling arena. After years of counseling, It is rare for me to loose a couple to divorce, and with that result I'm eternally grateful. This is the irony of ironies considering my own marital experience.

I have discovered that techniques, strategies, and improvement practices certainly have a place in relationships. However, it is more important to understand the Biblical core of man and woman, Christ-based principles, and empowerment.

It is at this point, I understand those persons without such a basis may tune-out the remainder of this exercise. However, to those who remain, you will discover the beginnings of a powerful truth.

Understanding Rebels and Tyrants: The Bible records that God created man, both male and female as co-equal rulers with dominion over every possession of the earth. Woman was not created as an after-thought or as if God forgot her. I personally reject the translation that she was a mere compatible helper on both grammatical and contextual grounds. Grammatically, the word translated helper is used several time where it is related to God as a savior or champion (Exo. 18:4; Deu 33:7; Psa. 33:20; Psa 70:5).

Secondly, when God decreed the female's punishment for sin, God stated that her husband would "rule" her. Therefore, prior to sin her husband did not rule her. Finally, man (i.e., male and female) was made in the very image of God, and in His likeness. The Bible records a singular and co-equal God-head comprised of the Father, Son, and the Holy Spirit. Similarly, man is a singular creation with co-equal genders. Only after sin, does headship become an issue.

Concerning man, both male and female, they were provided every "creature" comfort and need with only one prohibition. They were not to eat from the tree of the knowledge of good and evil (Gen. 2:17). However, the female was deceived, and she decided to rebel by violating this singular prohibition. Continuing with her purpose as co-equal and co-ruler, she also gave the fruit to her husband who was not deceived. The Bible records that he also consumed the fruit (Gen. 3:1-6).

As the story unfolds, God begins His rhetorical inquiry. Obviously, the male version of man was created first. Doubtlessly, for this reason, he is questioned initially about the transgression. Thereafter, the male identifies the female as the culprit. Most see this as the first excuse or blame. And who is to argue with such a point? Although the male's participation was undeniable, there was irony in the male's disclosure to God, "it was the woman you gave me." Most of us shrink at the thought that the male also includes God as partially at fault. Strikingly, God responds by proceeding to the woman. He questions her about her participation. Clearly, God already knew the full extent of their participation, but he provides due process.

Consequently, the female falls from co-ruler to one who has to seek the affection of the remaining ruler, her "husband." God pronounces, "your desire shall be to your husband, and he shall rule you" (Gen. 3:16). God's administration of this condition is in obvious response to her decision to rebel and misappropriate her position as co-ruler. It is understood that this specter of rebellion is going to remain with her, and she will encounter a tyrannical husband who will never willingly accept her advice without scrutiny and scorn. Afterwards, she'll be confronted with an innate spirit of rebellion, and the male becomes a dominating force with innate bitterness toward her.

God precedes the pronouncement against the male with the clause, "because you listened to the voice of your wife and have eaten from the tree…" Clearly, God recognizes the participation by both parties. The statement indicates the woman's leadership in the rebellion and the man's collaboration.

As created, the union between male and female was designed to be completely transparent and homogenous, but Man's (male and female) insurrection against the counsel of God incorporated the core elements of natural enemies. Now, they would be two people drawn to each other as designed, but possessing self-destructive, and relationally-destructive characteristics.

As progenitors of all subsequent generations, the built-in tension was set. Every person, male and female would possess the same characteristics. Throughout history, it is as if the female is attempting to recapture her prior state of authority, while the male continues to limit and dominate her to the degree possible.

Interestingly, cultures extolling autonomy, self-reliance, and independence with tolerant divorce laws have high divorce rates. This is not an effort to recommend tougher divorce laws as an answer. Instituting stricter divorce codes will not lead Christian couples to fulfill the purpose God has in their lives as joint heirs.

Excluding spiritual forces of evil, I have found in my Christ-based counseling practice, the core relational problem in Christian marriages is male tyranny and female rebellion.

The apostles, Paul and Peter provide specific principles in line with Jesus (Christ-o-centric) teachings. Considering male and female beginnings as discussed above, it is clear why the Lord through the instruction of his apostles outline key marital principles as follows:

Spirit-filled Principle: Christ-based principles for living cannot be implemented in the believers' life without the power, presence, and fullness of the Spirit. Most Christian couples, male and female do not invest in practices designed to develop spiritual fortitude. Yes, they attend church, and most couples confess the Lord Jesus Christ, and there is no doubt about their sincerity.

However, given the incredible pressure on Christian relationships, and the spiritual forces of darkness at work, a salvation confession marks the "beginning" of the battle to live victorious personal and relational lives. The Lord did not leave us without sound instructions concerning the preparation required to live victorious lives.

The Need for Spirit-fullness: Colossians, Chapter 3 and Ephesians, Chapter 5 identify the key component for a Christ-based marital union, and any other Christ-based purpose in the believer's life. Colossians 3:16-19, and Ephesians: 6:18-25 cite spirit-fullness as the key requirement, and provide demonstrations of spirit-fullness. You will notice that both demonstrations incorporate characteristics of the wife and husband respectively.

Most theologians agree that Colossians was written before Ephesians. So, Colossians 3:16-19 is presented first. Here, Paul uses the term "let the word of Christ dwell in you richly." Paul continues with the evidence of the word of Christ dwelling richly within the believer as follows: 1. Believers who teach and admonish one another with songs and hymns. 2. Believers who sing to one another with thankfulness. 3. Believers who do all in the name of Jesus. 4. Wives who submit to their husbands. 5. Husbands who love and who are not bitter toward their wives.

Later, Paul writes similar principles to the Ephesians. Instead of using the term, "let the word of Christ dwell in you richly," Paul states, "do not be filled with wine…but be filled with the spirit."

Clearly, "spirit-fullness," and the "word of Christ dwelling richly" are synonymous terms. This fact will be illustrated in more detail later. The demonstrations of spirit-fullness in a believer are summarized in verses 19 through 25 as follows: 1. Believers who speak to one another in songs and hymns. 2. Believers who always give thanks. 3. Believers who submit to one another 4. Wives who submit to husbands. 5. Husbands who love their wives as Christ loved the Church.

DEMONSTRATIONS or EVIDENCE

Spirit-fullness (Ephesians 6:19-25)	Word Dwelling Richly (Colossians 3: 16-19)
v. 19 Believers who speak to one another in songs and hymns	v. 16. Believers who teach and admonish one another with songs and hymns
v. 20 Believers who always give thanks	v. 16b Believers who sing with thankfulness
v.21 Believers who submit to one another	v. 17 Believers who do all in the name of Jesus…
v. 22 Wives who submit to husbands	v. 18. Wives who submit to their husbands
v. 25 Husbands who love their wives as Christ loved the church…	v. 19 Husband who love their wives and are not bitter toward them.

Notice in both cases that among social relationships, Paul identifies the wife and husband as persons who demonstrate "spirit-fullness." The demonstration of the spirit-filled wife is that she submits. Only a spirit-filled wife can make submission a practical reality in her life. Otherwise, her relationship with her husband is more oriented toward usurping headship. She's more inclined to battle for authority and control.

It is not a mystery why God's word addresses the woman first and at length concerning being subject to her husband. Concerning the husband and wife, rebellion began with the female, and continues to be a core challenge for most women to overcome.

Peter adds a remarkable statement concerning a woman's spirit and how to please God. Comparing investments in outer appearance to the value of inner beauty Peter states, "

but let it be the hidden person of the heart, with the imperishable quality of a gentle and quiet spirit, which is precious in the sight of God." This is true for any person male or female, but it is a particularly noteworthy characteristic of a spirit-filled wife.

However, the principal responsibility for the relationship is squarely on the spirit-filled husband. Love including submissiveness is his primary trait (Ephesians 6:21,25). Otherwise, he will attempt to dominate, control and oppress his wife. Notice the admonition in Colossians 3:19. Paul adds, "don't be bitter toward them." Again, this prohibition is in direct alignment with the males' innate and original tendency to rule his wife.

No man can love his wife as Christ loved and died for the Church without the fullness of the Spirit.

Today, couples reveal the difficulty of trying to uphold such principles in their relationships. Well, this is not new. It was a difficult issue when Paul wrote these principles two thousand years ago. Notice the additional explanation that he gives the Ephesians concerning the relationship responsibilities.

When writing the Colossians in verses 3:16-19, he gives brief statements. Wives be subject to your husbands...Husbands love your wives and do not be embittered against them. Later, when he writes the Ephesians he provides more detail (Ephesians 5:22 -33).

Obviously, Paul witnessed the need for additional instructions. The same responses that we hear today were apparent more than two thousand years ago. These instructions to both the husband and wife were difficult to accept.

Herein lies the watershed truth of Biblical revelation concerning male-female relationships. The rebellious nature of the female, and tyrannical nature of the male has always been an issue since the day of evil in the Garden. It is not an accident or coincidental that Paul leads into his guidance on the core characteristics of the wife and husband with terms such as, "be filled with the spirit," and "let the word of Christ dwell in you richly." Paul recognized that these are key to the spiritual purpose, life, strength and personal fulfillment of all relationships.

How can a husband, wife, or any other believer become spirit-filled? Couples and individual's alike who desire to fulfill the Lord's purpose in their relationships, desire to be spirit-filled.

Recognizing the enemy of all social relationships: Paul follows his instructions concerning spirit-fullness, and social relationships with a startling disclosure in the following Chapter. No Biblical writer had ever uncovered the sinister operation of spiritual darkness and evil in such graphic detail as Paul offers in Ephesians, Chapter 6. Recognizing the spiritual forces' of darkness efforts to destroy every social relationship, Paul uncovered this diabolic operation so that every believer would prepare to win the ongoing assaults. After Paul concludes his demonstrations of spirit-filled believers in social relationships (Ephesians 6:1-9), Paul identifies the adversary to spirit-fullness. He further states, "be strong in the Lord and the power of His might. Put on the full armor of God that you may be able to stand firm against the schemes of the devil."

Notice the instruction to "put on." Here, the believer is instructed to act. Paul continues by outlining a number of necessary acts in order to withstand the assaults of this invisible and powerful foe (Ephesians 6:10-15). First, believers must stand (vs. 14). They do not stand in their own strength, but they stand as persons who have been purchased by the blood and righteousness of Jesus. They stand on the truth of the gospel of peace (vs. 15). They recognize that a crumbling relationship is not the work of their spouse, but the result of spiritual wickedness. Clearly, it was Paul's objective that believers target spiritual evil as the culprit, and not spouses, fellow-believers, and others.

These are my very words in counsel. When a counselee states, "my spouse has asked am I leaving or you"? When it is clearly a situation where no one should be moving I respond, "stand." Notice, believers stand on the gospel of peace. Peace comes from the fact that spirit-filled believers know they are going to win. Come what may, spirit-filled believers WIN! (Phil 4:6-7; Rom.8:28-29). This Biblical truth is what gives peace in the midst of difficult circumstances.

Three Keys to Spirit-fullness and Marital health: Once a spouse or spouses know that their position against evil is to stand, they have further acts to employ. Now, Paul combines an unbeatable threesome in verses 16 through 18.

1. Faith "Fullness" v. 16: He identifies "faith" as an element, which overcomes every assault of Satan. Regardless of how dire the circumstances appear, spouses must believe that the Lord is operating through their marred and stained relationships. People of faith look beyond their frustration, sense of loss, pain and agony to a time of deliverance and resurrection.

2. Word "Fullness" v. 17: Paul follows the appeal to faithfulness with the source of faithfulness, God's word. Where feelings, presumptions, and appearances dash hopes and desires, God's word is the immovable and impenetrable guarantee. God's word becomes an offensive weapon in the believers' life. Isaiah the prophet said it best, "No weapon that is formed against thee shall prosper; and every tongue that shall rise against thee in judgment thou shalt condemn. This is the heritage of the servants of the Lord, and their righteousness is of me, saith the LORD" (Isa. 54:17). There is no doubt that the Lord's word through the prophet to His people has more significance today, and the weapons formed by spiritual principalities are those, which are defeated.

Earlier, I discussed Paul's usage of two terms, "spirit-filled" and "word of Christ dwelling richly." Paul shows the relationship between the spirit and God's word. He encourages the believer to take the sword of the spirit, which is the word of God. The "knock-out" instrument of the spirit is God's word. This is further contextual evidence of the synonymous relationship between spirit-fullness and the word of Christ dwelling richly.

Given faith, and God's word, Paul adds the final and most therapeutic agent of the three, prayer. Spouses must have consistent and targeted prayer lives concerning their relationships.

3. Prayer "Fullness" v. 18: Concerning desires, which involve any area of life James said it best, "you have not, because you ask not....you ask and do not receive because you ask with wrong motives."

Spouses need to request in prayer the principles God desires for them. The combination of asking for what God desires in one's life, AND asking the way Jesus instructed guarantees God's approval. We know he hears and answers our petitions (I John 5:14-15).

Husbands need to ask the Lord to make them husbands according to Ephesians Chapter 6, and Colossians, Chapter 3. Wives need to ask the Lord to make them wives according to Ephesians Chapter 6, and Colossians, Chapter 3. Notice how the husband focuses on his own need, and the wife does likewise. Their spirit-filled characteristics do not depend on mutual performance. Their spirit-filled characteristics depend on faith, God's principles in His word, and persistent prayer in their lives.

When I ask troubled couples, "are you praying about your situation"? They usually answer, yes. However, when I provide illustrations of what Jesus meant by prayer, rarely do they respond so positively.

I do not desire to discourage persons who pray on the move. However, praying on the move, or where distractions readily occur do not rise to the standard of prayer set by Jesus. There are two ways Jesus instructed his disciples about prayer. He did so by word and deed. A powerful prayer life requires adherence to the principles, which Jesus demonstrated about prayer. First, Jesus spoke of the "closed door" prayer (Matt. 6:1-6). Likewise, Jesus would seek quiet and remote areas when he desired quality time with his Father. Mountains, gardens, and seaside retreats were his favorite places for personal time with his Father. It is no mystery that in history's darkest hour before His death, Jesus and his friends headed toward a quiet place. Then once they arrived, he further separated himself from his friends (Matt. 26:36; Mark 14:32).

Jesus and the three stages of prayer: Jesus leaves the majority of his disciples at one area of Gethsemane. He takes others further with him. Finally, he parts from these remaining disciples where he is completely alone (Matt. 26:36-39, Mark 14:32-35). All of the groups should have been praying. The Gethsemane experience illustrates three stages of prayer. I refer to these as "porch" or preparation stage, "sanctuary" or general stage, and "holy of holies" stage.

Porch or Preparation stage: This is the stage where we begin by praising and thanking God for who He is. We praise Him for His greatness, majesty, and works in creation. Thanking Him for the seen and unseen manifestations of His hand.

Sanctuary or General stage: This is the stage where we continue our prayer with petitions for others. We make requests for our nation, employers, ministries, and significant others.

Holy of Holies or Intensive stage: This is the stage where we pray for the things most dear to our lives. We pray for our personal lives. We make our personal requests before him concerning His preeminence and will in our lives. We pray for the salvation and care of our spouses, our children and other personal concerns.

It is also a noteworthy parallel between these three stages of prayer and the Old Testament tabernacle or temple, which included an entry way or porch, sanctuary, and holy place.

Spirit-fullness requires finding quality time each day to get before our Father. Among the many things Jesus said about prayer, two illustrations stand vividly in my mind each time I pray. They are both found in Luke, Chapters 11 and 18.

The first in Luke 11:5-8, is a scenario Jesus presents to his disciples. Jesus explained that at midnight a disciple asked a neighborhood friend for bread to feed a visiting friend. The neighborhood friend refused because he and his family were sleep. Jesus concludes that the slumbering friend would arise and provide the bread because of the persistency of the friend making the request.

Several points are clear. The two persons, the one requesting and the other sleeping had a pre-existing friendship. Likewise, believers have a greater relationship with God. Secondly, there is significance in the time of the request. The request was made at midnight. In the midst of family crisis, I can recall that my most trying and emotional times occurred during the midnight. It was as if morning would never arrive. Often the greatest needs occur when no one else is available, or they are busy with the affairs of their own lives.

The original language of the New Testament is Greek. A term for the action of a verb that is complete is "punctilliar." "Jesus is risen" is punctilliar. This means that the action of a subject comes to a point, period, or destination and does not continue. The action is complete. Conversely, Jesus identifies persistency as a necessary factor of prayer. Prayer by definition is continuous or it is not prayer, and some objects of prayer are ongoing. As long as we have parents, siblings, children, fellow-believers and spouses, prayer will be continuous on their behalf.

Remember, prayer is not punctilliar. Prayer is continual. A generation ago in my culture, old saints would say, "I'm sending up my timber." They understood that a great fire requires plenty of fuel. And victorious lives in Christ require on-going prayer.

Jesus concludes His instruction on prayer by providing a comparison between man and God's abilities to answer requests.

Most spouses or parents go to great lengths to respond to the needs of their loved ones. The best earthly parents do so with ill-motives, inconsistencies, and failures. Jesus compares earthly parents with their faults to our [perfect] heavenly Father. The obvious conclusion is that God will far exceed earthly parents with His care for His children (Luke 11:11-13). Jesus insists that we pray continually, and our heavenly Father will provide.

The second illustration is found in Luke 18:1-8. The parable begins with a purpose statement (v. 1). The expressed purpose of the parable was to demonstrate that believers should always pray and not give up. Here, Jesus tells the story of a judge who was not intimidated by God or man. No one could manipulate, trick, or pressure him with wealth, power, or religious influence. A widow representing the weakest person in society pleads for the judge's protection from an adversary. Initially, the judge was not moved at all by her plea. However, the woman's consistency and determination made the judge ponder his initial decision. He ultimately reasons that he is not intimidated by God or man, but the woman has caused him to reconsider his position. He granted her plea to stop her from wearing him out. Jesus concludes the parable by stating, "hear what the unrighteous judge said. Shall not God bring justice for His children who cry to him day and night."

The combination of prayer consistency, prayer persistency, and prayer with deep emotional compassion for one's cause moves God to action.

Relational Recovery: Paul's words ring clear concerning recovering from outbursts, disagreements, disappointments, misunderstandings, and other events causing discord:

Be angry, and yet do not sin; do not let the sun go down on your anger, and do not give the devil an opportunity (Ephesians 4:26-27).

Unsettling events and disputes will occur between couples. Respective spouses must recognize error, and think through the situation. They need to ask the Lord to rescue them, and take the necessary actions to repair the situation. Therefore, the best way to recover from a major dispute is to (RPA) recognize, pray, and apologize.

Excluding insolent behavior described below, spiritual leadership places this responsibility on the male.

A Sincere Apology: A sincere apology is one without conditions. "I apologize that I did this", or "did not do that." If an apology is bound with all kinds of conditions and fault redirected toward the spouse, then it is not a sincere apology. It will probably make the matter worse.

When an Apology Requires Action: Depending on what the event involved, more than an apology may be in order. If the event rises to the level of a personal attack, physical acts, physical abuse, name-calling, infidelity, and other abuses, a promise to seek counseling or recommended action is in order. Additionally, such acts may invalidate one's confession as a believer if the act or acts violate the Principal Care doctrine (see Marriage, Divorce, and the Believer).

The Spouse You Gave Me: There are occasions when a believing spouse is insolent. The spouse is unrepentant, and continues to hurt, mistreat, offend, and otherwise violate the marriage relationship. This type of issue is addressed at length in Marriage, Divorce and the Believer. Nevertheless, this alternative is provided in addition to those steps listed in Marriage, Divorce and the Believer. Similar to resolving matters between believers in the Church, the insolent spouse must be informed about the transgressions. If the behavior continues, Christ-based counseling should be arranged. If the offender does not agree to counseling, the offended spouse should turn the spouse over to the Lord for reproof. However, this is the most severe decision. A spouse is asking the Lord to correct and/or reprove the insolent loved one. Spouses making such a request should be prepared for whatever the Lord deems necessary to correct the behavior.

Spirit-filled Husbands and Wives: Given, spouses who rely on the Spirit's operation in their lives, they will be transformed to a relationship, which represents Christ and the Church. They no longer act as rebels and tyrants toward each other. They have Christ-based unions designed to demonstrate the power of Jesus Christ in their relationships.

Recommended CBC Exercises:

    Process of Being Made Whole
    Marriage, Divorce and the Believer
    Because You Listened to the Voice of Your Wife

Scripture Versions

King James Version, KJV
New American Standard Bible, NASB

1. What is written in volumes?

2. What is more important than relational techniques, strategies, and improvement practices?

Understanding Rebels and Tyrants

3. What book records facts about the creation of man?

4. Who were co-rulers?

5. Was woman an after-thought?

6. Why does the study reject the translation that woman was a mere compatible helper?

7. 7. Prior to sin, did male rule the female?   Explain.

8. What was provided for the male and female?

9. Once the female was deceived what did she decide to do?

10. Why did God question the male first?

11. Who did the male blame for the transgression?

12. Did God already know the full extent of their sin?

13. As the result of their sin, what does God pronounce concerning the female's participation?

14. What kind of spirit is going to remain with her, and who will never willingly accept her advice without scrutiny and scorn?

15. Before his pronouncement against the male, what did God give as the reason?

16. Who lead the rebellion against God?

17. Who collaborated?

18. What did man's insurrection against God incorporate into the relationship?

19. What would these two people possess?

20. Concerning men and women, what is evident throughout history?

21. What is the core relational problem in Christian marriages?

Spirit-filled Principle:

22. What cannot be experienced without the power, presence, and fullness of the Spirit?

23. Do most Christian couples, male and female, invest in practices designed to develop spiritual fortitude?   Explain.

24. What marks the beginning of the battle to live victorious Christian lives?

25. Did the Lord leave us without sound instructions concerning the preparation required to live victorious lives?

The Need for Spirit-fullness:

26. What two passages of Scripture identify the key component for a Christ-based marital union, and any other Christ-based purpose in the believer's life?

27. What is the term that Paul uses in Colossians 3:16-19?

28. Give the 4 demonstrations of the term used in Colossians 3:16-19?

29. What term does Paul use in Ephesians 5:19-25 that is the same as "word of Christ dwelling richly."?

30. What are the 5 demonstrations in Ephesians 5:19-25?

31. Among social relationships, what two persons are used to demonstrate spirit-fullness?

32. What is the demonstration of a spirit-filled wife?

33. What is she inclined to do if she is not spirit-filled?

34. Why do scriptural texts address the woman first?

35. What characteristic about a spirit-filled woman is precious in the sight of God?

36. Who bears the principal responsibility for the relationship?

37. Love including _____ is the male's primary trait?

38. If the husband is not spirit-filled, what will he attempt to do concerning his relationship with his wife?

39. Is it a new thing that couples reveal the difficulty of upholding such principles as wives submitting, and husbands loving their wives as Christ gave Himself for the church?   Explain

40. Why does Paul give more instructions to the Ephesians than he does to the Colossians concerning husbands and wives?

41. What is the watershed truth of Biblical revelation concerning the male-female relationship?

42. What is key to the spiritual purpose, life, strength and personal fulfillment of all relationships?

Recognizing the Enemy of All Social Relationships

43. What does Paul offer in Ephesians, Chapter 6 that had never been uncovered in such graphic detail?

44. Why did Paul uncover this?

45. Did Paul identify the adversary of spirit-fullness?

46. What is every believer instructed to put-on?

47. What must believers do first?

48. And what do believers stand on?

49. Is a crumbling relationship the work of a spouse?

50. Who did Paul want the believer to target as the culprit for a crumbling relationship?

51. Where does peace come from?

52. Come what may, what is the outcome for believers?

Three Keys to Spirit-fullness and Marital Health

53. What is the first key to spirit-fullness and marital health?

54. What must spouses believe about the Lord, and where He is operating concerning their marital relationship?

55. People of faith are able to look beyond what?

56. What is the source of faithfulness?

57. Compared to feelings, presumptions, and appearances, how does God's word perform?

58. What kind of weapon does God's word become in the believer's life?

59. What did Isaiah the prophet state?

60. What weapons are defeated?

61. What is the knock-out instrument of the spirit?

62. After faith, and God's word, what is the most therapeutic agent of the three keys?

63. Concerning desires or needs, what did James say?

64. What do spouses need to request in prayer?

65. What guarantees God's approval?

66. What do husbands need to ask the Lord to make them?

67. What do wives need to ask the Lord to make them?

68. The husband focuses on the _____ spirit-filled need?

69. 69. The wife focuses on the _____ spirit-filled need?

70. Their spirit-filled characteristics depend on what three keys?

71. Does praying on the move, or where distractions readily occur satisfy the standard of prayer taught by Jesus?

72. What two ways did Jesus use to teach His followers about prayer?

73. What does a powerful prayer life require?

74. How did Jesus demonstrate the "closed door" prayer?

75. In History's darkest hour where did Jesus and His friends go?

Jesus and three stages of prayer

76. Once they arrived at Gethsemane, what should each group be doing?

77. The Gethsemane experience illustrates how many stages of prayer?

78. What happens in the Preparation Stage of prayer?

79. What happens in the Sanctuary Stage of prayer?

80. What happens in the Holy of Holies Stage of prayer?

81. These three stages are parallel to what Old Testament form?

82. What does spirit-fullness required each day?

83. Who gives the example of prayer in Luke 11:5-8?

84. After initially refusing to give his friend some bread for his friend's visitor, why did the slumbering friend get up and give his friend the bread?

85. Was the request for assistance made from one friend to another?

86. If the slumbering friend arose to help his friend, what can we conclude about God's willingness to provide for us?

87. What time was it when the request was originally made?

88. What does Jesus identify as a necessary factor of prayer?

89. After comparing our provisions for the persons we love, what is the obvious conclusion concerning God and our needs?

90. What is it that Jesus insists?

91. Who gives the example of prayer in Luke 18:1-8?

92. What was the expressed purpose of the parable in Luke 18:1-8?

93. What was the characteristics of the judge in the parable?

94. What did the widow represent in society?

95. What was the judge's initial decision concerning the woman's plea?

96. What was it about the widow that caused the judge to reconsider his initial decision?

97. Why did the unjust judge grant her request?

98. Comparing the unjust judge to our just God, what will God do?

99. What are the prayer characteristics of God's children?

100. What moves God to action?

Relational Recovery:

101. Concerning outbursts, disagreements, disappointments, misunderstandings and other similar events, what does Paul admonish believers to do?

102. Will unsettling events and disputes occur between couples?

103. What must spouses do to overcome their differences?

104. What is (RPA)?

105. Excluding insolent behavior, who has the primary responsibility for RPA?

106. What are the characteristics of a sincere apology?

107. When does an apology require additional action?

The Spouse Your Gave Me

108. Describe an insolent spouse?

109. Carefully describe the steps to take with an insolent spouse?

110. What other resource is available, which provides additional advice about insolent or unrepentant spouses?

Spirit-filled Husbands and Wives

111. What will happen with spouses who rely on the Spirit's operation in their lives?

Actual Christ-based Counseling Notes to a Family Concerning Families with Step-children, and Teenaged or Adult Children

The Children Issues

It takes time for the couple to become one flesh. They are "one" flesh, but they may not initially operate as one flesh. As they learn and mature with each other over time, they should begin to "become" one flesh in their ability to understand and work with each other. I emphasize "they should" here.

NOW, if you add other personalities to the "mix" such as children from a previous relationship, the time required for this "working" together to "become" one flesh is going to be extended indefinitely. There are a number of "variables" here, which determine when and how you will be able to "become" one flesh.

As an example, the age of a child is extremely important. Another factor is the length of time a new spouse was single with "his" or "her" offspring.

Other issues include ex-spouses or significant-others who are parents of the children, and interaction by friends and relatives.

If the children are younger (e.g., 1-7 years old), it is easier for a new spouse to be introduced and live with the "step" children. However, if the children are pre-teens and teenagers with personalities and habits already resident, the new relationship will be more challenging.

I have found in my experience that usually the new "spouses" can get along if it were not for the difficulty of "how" to deal with the children. As I mentioned, if they are real young, the problem is not as difficult as far as dealing with the children. However, even with younger children issues such as "discipline" (e.g., Who will do it? What discipline "patterns" will be used?), and similar practices must be thoroughly accepted by both spouses.

The new couple must consider what they hold to be objectionable behavior, and what will be done about it. It is an "excellent" rule of thumb to allow the "natural" parent to institute "corrections." Under circumstances where both parents are the natural parents of a child, I recommend that the parent who observed the behavior take the corrective action. However, in the step-parent situation with older children, generally, the step-parent should not institute the corrective action.

Again, this is particularly important with older children. A step parent who creates new policy and distrupts the flow children expect with the natural parent is going to be greeted with hostility. Children and parents have a "flow" in their home and relationships. Children understand how the parents respond to things they do. And children know who to approach in the family. Usually, a child approaches the parent believed to give the most desired result. An excellent Biblical example of this fact is in (Gen. 25:27 and following). Consider the lives and Jacob and Esau. Jacob was closer to his mother, and Esau was closer to his father.

When a new spouse is introduced, this "flow" gets disrupted. The children do not have the same access. This also happens if the new spouse begins without many demands, but "later" changes and begins to insist on certain demands.

Nevertheless, the natural parent "feels" the pressure from the disruption of the flow recognizing that it is making "his" or "her" natural children resentful. The natural parent feels the pressure of being between "spouse" and natural child. The step-parent "feels" he or she is not being supported by the "natural" spouse. And if they are believers the spouse who is the step-parent may remind the "spouse" with step-children that he or she is higher in God's order than the children. That is, the husband's or wife's desire should come before the children. Although it was Sarai's idea that Abram would conceive a child through her handmaiden, Sarai wanted Ishmael and his mother "excommunicated" from their presence. Apparently, this was not difficult for Sarai to demand, but it caused an extreme hardship for Abram who was the natural parent. Sarai's demand illustrates that she assumed her place as a higher priority than Abram's son. It was only after God directed Abraham to do as Sarai demanded that Abram found peace with Sarai's demand. Generally speaking, it is Biblically accurate that the man and woman become one flesh. However, in the "step-parent" situation, it is not a social or familial reality for some time (Gen. 16:1-6; 21:9-14). It is noteworthy that at this time in their relationship, Sarai is not the more spiritually mature Sarah yet. And Abram is not the more spiritually mature Abraham yet. So, any spouse expecting another spouse to repudiate or discard an offspring to any degree can expect an intense situation. There are circumstances where an offspring is so disruptive or dishonorable that even the natural parent is in complete agreement.

Understanding the Dynamics of One Flesh Compared to a Natural Child

Please note Gen. 2:23, "For this reason a man shall leave his father and mother and cling to his wife, and they shall become one flesh" (Gen 2:23, Matt 19:5, Eph 5:31). Notice the "man" leaves his father and mother, and "shall," become one flesh. How does this happen? Because women is bone of his bone, and flesh of his flesh, and woman is taken out of man. The goal "even" today is for the two to "become" one. Therefore, spiritually they are one-flesh or of the same order; but practically it may be some time before they operate as "one-flesh."

Yes, with the first man and woman they were "one" flesh. However, do not be fooled. As the result of sin's impact over the ages, we do not enter a "perfect" male-female relationship simply by "saying" vows. As with our walk with Jesus, this relationship of bone-to-bone and flesh-to-flesh develops over time. And although we are justified immediately upon accepting Jesus as savior, we become more like Jesus over time.

HOWEVER, with our natural children it is different. Notice the man leaves his father and mother and cleaves to his wife. Right? Here's another question. Who was he "cleaving" to before he is to "cleave" to his wife? The answer is simple. It is understood the man is "cleaving" to his parents. We must remember what causes the "cleaving." The man or child is literally, bone of his parent's bone and flesh of his parent's flesh.

So, now here comes a new spouse, who demands this "higher" order. Guess what? That new spouse can forget it. This new spouse has not "become" bone of bone and flesh of flesh, and this can be proven.

Children or a child of a natural parent is bone-of-bone and flesh-of-flesh by birth. Therefore, a spouse has entered a marital relationship where in fact, the children are higher order than the spouse. And this is the incredible crisis a natural parent feels when something is making this parent's natural-child unhappy, particularly if the natural-parent views the spouse's conduct as unwarranted.

Now, the step-children may appreciate and really like the step-parent, but it is not the same. Also, it is not necessary to have the same natural disposition toward step children. However, the same level of care, concern, and positive regard is imperative. There are times when step-parents exceed the positive care and concern for step-children exhibited by the natrual parent.

So, how do we work together in a marital situation. First, I would recommend to anyone with children to entertain having a "long" term engagement. This will allow the children to become grown and move. Or it will allow the children to know that eventually, the fiance will be the spouse. It provides a long period for everyone to become "intimately" familiar with each other. The prospective spouses "show" their absolute behavior and patterns from the beginning so the relationship can be discontinued or determined to be acceptable.

Discipline Patterns Considerations

Even parents who are both the natural parents of a child have difficulty deciding what will be the discipline pattern, and type of pattern. Most importantly, whatever decisions are made must be agreed by both parents. And disagreements should never be discussed before the child.

Nevertheless, concerning step-children, the natural parent is the key person. Typically, the natural parent is going to be more sensitive to discipline issues than the step-parent. Typically, the natural parent is more lenient and less forceful with discipline. Again, this may not be true in every case, but most often it is correct.

Therefore, when the behavior is clearly wrong, there can be no doubt that discipline must be administered. Repeated behavior must be met with increased application of corrective measures. Natural parents must insist on appropriate behavior, and they must apply clearly corrective measures. Step-parents must provide opportunity for improvement, and lean to caution more than criticism. However, when a step-parent identifies a lack of consistency, or improvement in a step-child's behavior the natural parent must view the matter as factually as possible.

Step-parents and Discipline

Natural parents should carefully observe, and clearly express their approach to discipline with the step-parent. Additionally, a natural-parent must not marry a person who cannot be trusted with disciplining a natural child. Any parent, whether natural or step parent who ignores regular and consistent discipline is seriously disabling the child (Hebrews 12: 5-8).

Identifying Inappropriate Behavior

Inappropriate behavior is behavior that will injure the child, or injure others. Injury can be physically, mentally, socially, or otherwise.
Disobedient behavior, argumentative demeanor, deceit, rudeness, and similar conduct is unacceptable. Correction should be commensurate with the degree of damage or potential for damage in the present or future.
Remember, children are being prepared for society in general. What parents may tolerate and allow may be met with retribution in society. Prepare the child for living when protective parents will not be available.

Final Word for Disciplining Step-Children

The older a child is, the greater the caution observed by the parents when administering discipline.
If you are going to interact in terms of discipline, you must interact

with the same discipline pattern as the natural parent, unless the natural parent agrees otherwise. And each time correction is required you must have the full consent of the natural parent or don't do it. This is very difficult. The natural parent must keep in mind the issues discussed in the topics in the aforementioned.

Now, this sounds like a lot of policy for dealing with children, but the damage, which results from not being on one accord can destroy a family.

Remember a simple principle as a spouse. The husband and wife are developing as bone of bone, or flesh of flesh, but the natural child in reality is bone of bone and flesh of flesh. And the natural child is far more acquainted with the manners and expectations of the natural parent.

Dealing with Chults and Adult Children

A difficult task as a parent is living with a "CHULT." A chult is a person who is somewhere between childhood and adulthood. Clearly, it is easier if you raised them all of their days. Even then, there can be days when it is unbelievable. We had some drama out of our oldest child, in her senior year; but even that was not "in your face" kinda stuff.

How We All Live Together (Adult Children)

Given prayer and leadership, they must be consistently placed in the position of "autonomy." Here's some things we do.

Usually, we don't cook for them (once a week we try to eat together, Sunday).

They maintain their own rooms, and help with common areas.

Tim cuts the lawn on Thursdays, or other days as requested.

Weekdays everyone is in by 10:00 p.m. or they call for any exception.

They call if their daily schedule changes.

Weekends, no staying out all night. I remind them of the dangers of being out after 2:00 a.m. Other than that it's their call.

Attend church (either service), Sunday School, and Bible Study.

Unless scholarshipped, they must go to work and school.

It's More About Accountability and Coordination than Control

When they call or inform us about a schedule change, they are not asking for permission. We treat them like adults. They are merely informing us that they will not be in as scheduled. Unless there is truly something pressing, I will always say, "o.k. I'll see you when you get in." If there is something they were supposed to do, I'll ask them about their "get-back" plan. It may take several reminders before they actually learn about adult accountability. Sometimes they think being an adult means they don't have to answer to anyone. As you know, this is not unique. Some adult spouses have the same behavior, and it becomes a serious problem. This is why I want our children to understand this principle as they develop.

If they meet opposition most of the time when they call with a schedule change, they will stop calling.

No More Parent/Kiddie Responsibilities

They also understand that at this point in their lives, we are helping them out of the kindness of our hearts. We desire to see them succeed, and we are providing the opportunity. We do not have the kind of responsibility as for "kiddies," such as feeding, clothing, homework, and similar activities. We may have commentary, insights, or suggestions about such things, but they have the decision making authority.

Here's A True Story About Allowing Autonomy

My son was dating this young lady for about 6 months. I had some serious reservations and concerns about this young lady. And I gave him the benefit of my insight. He was extremely hurt about my view of her situation, and he was angry for a couple of days. I was very clear with him that he could date her, or marry her if he so desired. I did not want him to go into a "complete" shell concerning girls he dated. He told the girl about our view. So she became reluctant to come over. I told him he could bring her over. This was not "personal" it was simply some "realities." I would tell her the same thing.

Anyway, to make sure that he understood that I meant it when I said he could continue to date her, occasionally I would ask, "how's Girly"? [using an alias here to protect the innocent]

It may have been a month or so later before the answer was, "ah Dad, I told her I need a little space."

If I would have insisted that he no longer see that girl, it would have been the worse thing I could have done.

More Rules…Means More Potential for Rebellion

My dad was one of the most anally retentive guys you could ever meet. When he was in the house, it was like walking on eggshells. I simply tried to stay away from him. It's shameful, but for me and my brothers it was like being liberated when he was in the streets chasing women, gambling and drinking, sometimes for days at a time. We couldn't enter the kitchen, turn the T.V. channel, or play the stereo without permission. And if he was there we weren't going to ask. And don't dare ask him for any money. It was like living behind the Red Curtain. And my father never, ever, said, "son, I love you." I never had a conversation with him until I was an adult. Everything was commands, "do this" or "why did you do that?" A slap upside the head was always in order. Sometimes he would just look at me like I was an alien. Sometimes a look says it all. My dad took me to the movies, one time. He played catch with me, one time. He came to one of my baseball games, one time.

Nevertheless, it was a blessing to have him. He was an excellent model of how NOT to be a father. Lord willing, I'll wheel chair him to church on Sunday (Father's day). The endearing love he never gave to me, I give to him. Hey, if it wasn't for JESUS!

Anyway, family members have complete autonomy of the common areas of the home (e.g., kitchen, family, exercise, library, etc.).

Watch Out for Mixed Messages

As I look back on it, I can say my dad was consistent. He never said, "son I love you," and his policy within the home was consistent. He made you feel like he did not want you there. It was like having to crawl at the master's feet for the slightest request. Conversely, we can say, "son or daughter, I love you." But if our policies within the home do not match-up with the words, we can save the, "I love you."

Every Man's Castle

I'm only sharing what I believe to be Godly counsel. We are not all equipped similarly, and thank God. However, there are principles, which are universal. Regardless of who the parents are, there's no greater parental model than our heavenly Father.

Punishing Adult Children

I would not advise anyone to punish adult children. A parent is more likely to insult and infuriate them more than anything else if one attempts to punish them. Adults share, admit, confess, and further communicate to resolve issues. When I'm disappointed, I will tell them so. This is what Jesus demonstrates working with His followers.

If we reach an impasse where there is an attitude, conduct, or behavioral problem that continues, it's Luke 15 time.

Luke 15 Time

You have clearly established "opportunity" and a "place" for your son to get turned around. It is a matter of public "testimony" with more than two or three witnesses that you have, and continue to provide what's necessary for him.

What James Dobson calls tough love, I prefer to call Luke 15 Time (Luke 15:11-24). It is one of the most difficult "calls" in the world to withhold support, expel, or excommunicate a loved one. The age of the offspring does not matter here.

The Scripture is extremely clear about the prohibition and outcome of a dishonorable son (e.g., Due. 21:18-22). Regardless of your son's background, the principle remains.

This is one reason why the parable of the prodigal son almost had to be just that, a "story." No one in real life would dare dishonor his father in such an overt fashion during that timeframe. The Pharisees would dishonor their parents covertly, but not outwardly. Jesus tells what is the most outrageous account of a son who dishonors his father in the most horrendous fashion. A son who would do such a thing would have to leave his country. He would be an outcast to his 20th generation cousin and most distant friend of the family. Lawfully, he could be stoned to death.

So as you know, the boy leaves his country. By the way, the father out-of-his love and wisdom, GIVES the boy the possessions/heirlooms the boy requested.

The boy is "having a ball" in the beginning. He's the life of the party with plenty of money to throw around, BUT famine strikes! You can imagine, the listeners are nodding their heads as Jesus continues with the story. They are thinking, "A-ha the boy is about to get what he had coming to him."

Eventually, the boy's circumstances (e.g., famine, labor, piggish existence) causes him to think differently. In Christ-based Counseling we call this, "PRODIGAL MOTIVATION." Finally, he comes to himself.

There's no indication that the Father goes after his son. There's no indication that the Father sent his son money. But, there can be no doubt that the father loves the boy.

Among other things this is principally a parable about LOVE.

However, we know the conciliatory truths about this story. One fact is that if the father sends support to his son in the foreign land, the boy would never come to himself. Most children do not appreciate the value of their parents until they are on their own.

Another conciliatory truth is the boy's spirit of repentance. Notice, he changes direction. He turns from his own will, and begins to look toward his father (vss. 17-19). I have a basic rule, which says, "Forgiveness without repentance, leads to sin without an end."

Before we are saved, we must admit our sinful condition, and after we are saved we must confess our sin. Even God does not forgive us, if we do not come to grips with our errors. This is an extremely important principle to practice or else our love will become irresponsible, and completely inconsistent with God's love.

Caution Flag

Interestingly, adults in general have difficulty admitting fault, and find it particularly difficult saying, "I apologize." So sometimes they apologize by a demonstration of behavior, and not necessarily words. So this could be your son's practice.

Nevertheless, if your message of love is consistent with your policy for living in your household, then it sounds like Luke 15 Time "may" have arrived.

Only you, and your wife can determine when that time has arrived. Love ya. Praying for ya! Doc.

Printed in the United States
137068LV00001B/43/A